pends on the meridians 〔...〕
ly and the limbs externa〔...〕
systems of the human b〔...〕
of the body. With the F〔...〕
nify all the organs and tissues of the human body, including the Six
Fu organs, the five sense organs, the nine orifices, the four limbs
and the bones, and through the effect of Qi, Blood and Body Fluid,
the integrated activities of the human body are carried out.

Under the guidance of the concept of wholism, TCM holds that
the human body maintains its physiological balance through the
functional activity of each of the Zang Fu organs and tissues as well
as the coordination and restriction of these organs and tissues. Besides, TCM places emphasis on the wholism when analyzing pathological mechanism of disease, or the wholistic reflection of a local
disease, and the relations between the local disease and the system-
atic one. In other words, it stresses both the directly related organs
or meridians of disease and the influence of these organs and meridians on the other. In the treatment of disease, TCM also stresses
that a proper therapeutic principle should be one that is made based
on the concept of wholism.

(2) Unity between man and nature: Man lives in nature where
exists the necessary conditions for man's survival, and nature exerts
its influence directly or indirectly on the human body, leading to its
corresponding changes. This kind of influence mainly lies in changes
of the seasons and climates, day and night and geographical conditions.

① Influence of seasonal and climatic changes on the human body:
The climate is warm in spring, hot in summer, wet in long-summer, dry in autumn and cold in winter. Influenced by the different
climates, creatures exhibit such changes as generating in spring,
growing in summer, becoming mature in long summer, astringing in
autumn and hiding in winter. Without exception, man also shows
such changes under the influence of different climates of different
seasons. For example, it is hot in summer, correspondingly, Yang
Qi of the human body goes to the exterior of the body, which leads

to relaxation of the skin and muscles and the ensuing polyhidrosis and scanty urine. In winter, it is cold, so Yang Qi of the human body hides in the interior, leading to closing of the skin and the resultant polyuria and little sweating.

The adaptive ability of the human body to the natural environments has its own limitation. When the climates in the four seasons change so rapidly as to exceed the adaptive ability of the human body, or when the adaptive ability of the human body is lowered and fails to correspond to the changes of the natural environments, disease will occur. As the climatic conditions in different seasons are different, different common or popular diseases will develop in different seasons. Aggravation or attack of some chronic disease is also related to violent change of weather or altering of seasons.

② Influence of day, night, morning and dawn on the human body: Although changes of the temperature in the morning, evening, day and night are not so obvious as these of the four seasons, they have certain influence on the human body. The physiological activities of the human body must be correspondent to the vissicitude of Yin and Yang in the different periods of a day. That is, Yang Qi of the human body tends to go outwards to the exterior in the day time and inwards to the interior at night. In most cases, diseases tend to be mild in the day time and severe at night.

③ Influence of the geographical conditions on the human body: Difference of the climatic conditions, geographical conditions and living habits in different regions also influence the human body to some extent. For example, it is hot and wet in South-China, so people living there usually have loose striae of muscles and are prone to suffer from disease caused by Damp Heat or that marked by convulsion; it is dry and cold in the North-China, so people living there usually have a closed striae of muscles and are more likely to suffer from disease marked by cold limbs or abdominal distention.

Man and nature are both opposite and unified. All the physiological and pathological phenomena of the human body are influenced by the natural environments. So, doctor must analyze the interconnections between the external environment and the internal changes of

Essentials of Traditional Chinese Medicine

Written by Ouyang Bing
Gu Zhen
Translated by Lu Yubin

Shandong Science and Technology Press

First Edition 1996
ISBN 7—5331—1843—X

Essentials of
Traditional Chinese Medicine

Written by	Ouyang Bing
	Gu Zhen
Translated by	Lu Yubin
Editor in charge	Zhong Pengjun

Published by Shandong Science and Technology Press
16 Yuhan Road, Jinan, China 250002
Printed by Shandong Dezhou Xinhua Printing House
Distributed by China International Book Trading Corporation
35 Chegongzhuang Xilu, Beijing 100044, China
P. O. Box 399, Beijing, China
Printed in the People's Republic of China

Preface

This is one volume of *The Series of Traditional Chinese Medicine for Foreign Readers*.

Traditonal Chinese medicine (TCM) is a complete theoretical system with well developed concepts and theories as well as rich clinical experience. This book, aiming at introduction to the basic theories and concepts of TCM, consists of eight parts. Part one is a brief introduction to the general conditions of TCM, including the development of TCM and its basic features; part two covers the philosophic concepts and theories that have deeply influenced the formation and development of the TCM theories, such as Yin Yang theory and Five Elements theory; part three, or the Visera-State theory in TCM, aims at introduction of the most important theories on human body in TCM, in which understanding of TCM about the internal organs and their physiological functions are concerned; part four deals with the Qi, Blood and Body Fluid which are regarded as the most basic substances constituting the human body and maintaining the normal physiological functions of the human body; part five introduces the meridian theory, which is a passageway through which Qi and Blood circulate through the human body; part six is an introduction to understanding of TCM on the etiological factors of diseases as well as occurrence of diseases; part seven is a part dealing with the analysis of TCM about the occurrence, development and changes of diseases; and part eight, the final part of this book, aims

1

at introduction of the basic ideas of TCM about the prevention and treatment of diseases.

This book is an essential book for foreign TCM learners and it may be used as a reference book for foreign TCM practitioners.

Compiler
July, 1996

Contents

Introduction

*T*raditional Chinese medicine (TCM) is a summation of the experience of the Chinese people in their long struggle against disease. As an important part of the great Chinese traditional culture, it has a history of several thousands years. Ever since its coming into being, it has made great contributions to the prosperity of the Chinese nation and the development of the world medicine.

Formation and Development of the Theoretical System of TCM

TCM is a subject dealing with the physiology and pathology of human body as well as the diagnosis, prevention and treatment of disease. It is a medicine with the concept of the wholism as its guiding thoughts, with the theory of Yin Yang and Five Elements as its theoretical tool, with the Zang Fu organs and the meridians as its theoretical basis, and with the Syndrome identification and corresponding treatment as its characteristics in diagnosis and treatment of disease.

1

It is generally accepted that the theoretical system of TCM was established during the period from the Warring States period to the Qin and Han Dynasties, marked by the accomplishment of the books *Huang Di Nei Jing* (The Yellow Emperor's Internal Classics), *Nan Jing* (The Difficult Classics) and *Shang Han Za Ning Lun* (Treatise on Febrile and Miscellaneous Disease).

During the Spring-autumn and Warring States period, rapid changes took place in Chinese society. The political thoughts, culture and economy shared great development and the academic thoughts became more and more rigorous. Right at this period, the first medical classic in the history of China, *Huang Di Nei Jing* (The Yellow Emperor's Internal Classics), emerged. This book summarized the medical achievements and the clinical experience before this period, described systematically the physiology and pathology of human body as well as the diagnosis, prevention and treatment of disease, setting up the theoretical system of TCM and Laying the basis of the development of TCM.

This book is now divided into two parts, *Su Wen* (The Plain Questions) and *Ling Shu* (The Miraculous Pivot). It involves the theory of viscera-state, meridians, pathogenesis, diagnostic methods, Syndrome identification, acupuncture therapy and decoction therapy. While it discusses the medical problems, it also makes deep exploration of a series of important philosophical problems at that time, such as the theory of Yin Yang, Five Elements, Qi, relations between man and nature and relations between body and spirit. Many achievements in this book are the most advanced in the world at that time. Even today, the main fundamental ideas and theoretical principles in TCM still take the description of the book as basis.

Nan Jing (The Difficult Classics), written before Han Dynasty by Qin Yueren, is also a book with rich contents. It covers almost every aspects of TCM such as the physiology and pathology of the human body and diagnosis and treatment of disease. It discussed and explained some medical problems mentioned in *Huang Di Nei Jing* (The Yellow Emperor's Internal Classics), thus it is a supplement to the book. *Nan Jing* (The Difficult Classics) and *Huang Di Nei Jing* (The Yellow Emperor's Internal Classics) are important theoretical basis guiding the clinical practice in later generations.

During the East and West Han Dynasties, rapid progress and development were seen in TCM. In the end East Han Dynasty, Zhang Zhongjing, a well-known physician, wrote a book named *Shang Han Za Ning Lun* (Treatise on Febrile and Miscellaneous Disease), based on the theories in *Huang Di Nei Jing* (The Yellow Emperor's Internal Classics) and *Nan Jing* (The Difficult Classics) through summarizing the medical achievements before him and that of his own. This book evolved afterwards into two books, *Shang Han Lun* (Treatise on Febrile Disease) and *Jin Gui Yao Lue* (Synopsis of the Prescriptions of Golden Chamber). *Shang Han Lun* (Treatise on Febrile Disease) created the principle of Syndrome identification in accordance with the six meridians, while *Jin Gui Yao Lue* (Synopsis of the Prescriptions of Golden Chamber) analyzed Syndromes based on the theory of Zang Fu organs. *Shang Han Za Ning Lun* (Treatise on Febrile and Miscellaneous Disease) is the first monograph that applies the Syndrome identification and corresponding treatment successfully in the history of TCM, and it provided a basis for the development of the clinical TCM.

Following *Huang Di Nei Jing* (The Yellow Emperor's Internal Classics) and *Shang Han Za Ning Lun* (Treatise on Febrile and Miscellaneous Disease), doctors of the later generations, in accordance with their clinical practice, developed TCM theory from different aspects. Wang Shuhe of the Jin Dynasty wrote a book entitled Maiagnosis systematically. In the Sui Dynasty, Chao Yuanfang finished the first monograph dealing with the etiology, pathology and Syndromes, *Zhu Bing Yuan Hou Lun* (Treatise on Etiology and Pathogenesis of Disease). Chen Wuze of the Song Dynasty put forward the famous "three categories of pathogen of disease" in his book *San Yin Ji Yi Bing Zheng Fang Lun* (Prescriptions Assigned to the Three Categories of Pathogenic Factors of Disease), and Qian Yi of the Song Dynasty created the method of Syndrome identification in accordance with the theory of Zang Fu organs. During the Jin

3

and Yuan Dynasties, there appeared different academic schools of medicine with their own different features, the most famous of whom are the schools represented by Liu Wansu who stressed the application of drugs of cool or cold nature, by Zhang Congzheng who put eliminating pathogens in the first place of treatment, by Li Gao who treated disease mainly by supplementing the Spleen and the Stomach, and by Zhu Danxi who paid special attentions to the treatment of disease with nourishing Yin. These four doctors are also known as the "four great doctors in the Jin and Yuan Dynasties." In the Ming Dynasty, Zhao Xianke, Zhang Jingyue, etc., suggested the importance of Mingmen in the human body. In the Ming and Qing periods, the theory of epidemic febrile disease occurred. And in the Qing Dynasty, Wang Qingren developed the theory of Blood Stasis as a pathogenic factor of disease. Doctors nowadays have also done multiple studies on the TCM theories.

The Materialistic and Dialectical Thoughts in TCM Theory

TCM was deeply influenced by the ancient philosophical thoughts in the formation of its theoretical system, and simple materialistic and dialectical thoughts goes through the whole theoretical system of TCM.

1. The materialistic thoughts

(1) Man being generated by combination of the heaven Qi and the earth Qi: TCM believes that Qi is the most basic substance substituting the material world. Life is the product of development of the material world to certain stage and is a process of constant development and change caused by the opposite and unity of Yin and Yang. Man is produced by the heaven Qi and the earth Qi, and essence Qi is the basic substance substituting the human body and maintaining its life activities. These ideas forms the idea of life being material,

which is a materialistic concept.

(2) Body and spirit being unable to be isolated: Based on the materialistic concept of nature, TCM stresses that body cannot be separated from the spirit. "Body" here refers to the body physique of the human beings, while "spirit" has many meanings, referring to ① the functional manifestations of the changes and motions of the things in the world and their intrinsic laws; ② the general outward manifestations of the life activities, and ③ the mental activities of the human body. In accordance with TCM, the body is the basis to produce the spirit, while the spirit can regulate and control the activities of the body. They depend on each other for their existence, and unity of the body and spirit is the main assurance of one's survival.

(3) Disease being able to be identified, prevented and treated: TCM seeks not only the causative factors of disease in nature, but also the intrinsic factors for the occurrence of disease in order to explain the pathologic changes of disease. So its concept of disease is materialistic. According to TCM, disease can be identified, prevented and treated. It suggests that preventive measures should be taken to prevent the occurrence of disease, and early diagnosis and treatment should be carried out once disease occurs.

2. The dialectical thoughts

In the light of TCM, everything in the world has common material source, and everything is closely related to and restricted by each other rather than isolated from each other nor immutable and frozen. Therefore, rich dialectical thoughts are developed in TCM.

TCM stresses that man is closely related to nature because he is a component of the world. Man is an organic unity in constant movement, in which the organs and tissues of the human body are closely related and influenced in either physiology or pathology. Meanwhile, TCM also stresses the intrinsic connection between the mental activities and the physiological activities and the counteraction of the spirit on the body.

In TCM, the law of occurrence and development of disease is recognized based on the concept of motion and interrelations with special emphasis placed on the different stages of disease, and the treatment aiming at the most fundamental causes of disease forms the main idea of treating disease.

The Basic Features of TCM

Under the guidance of the materialistic and dialectical thoughts, TCM developed its unique theoretical system through long period clinical practice. Compared with Western medicine, it has two basic features, the concept of wholism and the Syndrome identification and corresponding treatment.

1. The concept of wholism

Wholism refers to unity and integration. TCM believes that man is an organic unity in which the component parts of the human body are inseparable in structure, incorporated and supplemented in functions and influenced by each other in pathology. It also stresses that man is closely related to nature. Man maintains its normal life process by his passive adapting to nature and reforming nature. This kind of idea, unity of the internal and external environments and the unity of the human body itself, is known as the concept of wholism, which is carried out in almost every aspects of TCM, such as physiology, pathology, diagnostic methods, Syndrome identification and treatment.

(1) Man being an organic unity: The human body is composed of organs and tissues, which have their different functions. On one hand, these functions are component parts of the whole body's activities; on the other, they determine the unity and integration of the human body. In physiological conditions, these functions are related to each other and restricted by each other, maintaining the coordination and balance of the life activities, and in pathological conditions, diseases of the functions influence each other and can transmit from one to another. The unity of the body takes the Five Zang organs, which pair with the Six Fu organs, as their core, and de-

the body and adopt the therapeutic principles in accordance with the different seasons, locations and individuals in diagnosis and treatment of disease.

2. Syndrome identification and corresponding treatment

Syndrome identification and corresponding treatment serves as a basic principle of recognizing and treating disease in TCM. It is also a special method of studying and managing disease in TCM as well as one of the most basic features of TCM.

Syndrome is a summation of the essence of disease at certain stage of its development. It includes the location, cause, nature and the relation between pathogen and Vital Qi. As it reflects the essence of disease at a certain stage, it can illustrate the essence of disease more comprehensively, exactly and correctly than the symptoms. The so-called Syndrome identification refers to the process of determining a Syndrome of certain nature by analyzing the cause, nature and location as well as the relations between pathogen and Vital Qi of a disease through analyzing and synthesizing the data concerning the disease (including the symptoms and signs) gained through the four diagnostic methods of TCM, observing, smelling and auscultating, inquiring and palpating. Corresponding treatment is a therapeutic method determined based on the Syndrome identified. Syndrome identification is the prerequisite for the corresponding treatment, while the corresponding treatment is the means of treatment. Whether a correct therapeutic principle or method is adopted or not depends on whether a correct Syndrome identification is made or not, while whether the Syndrome identification is correct or not depends on examination of the therapeutic results. Therefore, Syndrome idemtification and corresponding treatment are a unity that cannot be separated. The both serve as the basic principle of diagnosis and treatment of disease in TCM. The process of Syndrome identification and corresponding treatment is in fact a process of diagnosing and treating disease.

It is imperative in TCM to carry out Syndrome identification in diagnosis and treatment of disease in order to determine the therapeutic principle and method, even if the disease has been identified.

Take common cold for example, proper therapeutic principle and method can be determined only when it is identified whether the disease is Wind Cold type or Wind Heat type, or whether it is still an exterior Syndrome or the pathogen has invaded the interior and transformed into Heat. Syndrome identification and corresponding treatment is different either from expectant treatment or from the treatment aiming at disease by using specific drugs.

As the most important law guiding diagnosis and treatment of disease in TCM, Syndrome identification and corresponding treatment can treat disease and Syndrome dialectically, for any disease may have different manifestations and different diseases may show the similar manifestations in clinic. For this reason, we may employ the method of treating the same disease with different methods or treating different diseases with the same method under the guidance of the principle of Syndrome identification and corresponding treatment. The so-called treating the same disease with different methods indicates that different therapeutic methods may be applied to one disease at its different stages as a result of the difference of the disease in the seasons and regions of its onset and the difference of patients' response. In a similar way, the so-called treating different disease with the same method indicates that different diseases may be treated with the same method as a result of occurrence of the same pathogenesis in their development. From this we can see that treatment of disease in TCM is based on the difference of pathogenesis of disease rather than the disease themselves. This is what is called treating the same Syndrome with the same method and treating different Syndromes with different methods. The essence of the Syndrome identification and corresponding treatment lies in that different contradictions in the development of disease should be solved differently.

Doctrines of Yin Yang and Five Elements

The doctrine of Yin Yang and Five Elements, a combined name for the theory of Yin Yang and that of Five Elements, is a theory used to understand the nature from the nature itself, explain the natural phenomena and explore the laws of nature. It is a world outlook and methodology in the ancient China. In the light of Yin Yang theory, the material world shows its occurrence, development and changes under the impetus of Yin Qi and Yang Qi, while according to Five Elements theory, wood, fire, earth, metal and water are the five kinds of most basic substances constituting the world, and all the phenomena of the material world lie in the motions and changes of the Five Elements.

Based on their long-standing clinical practice, the ancient Chinese doctors introduced the theory of Yin Yang and Five Elements into the medical field, so as to explain the physiological functions and pathological changes of the human body and to guide diagnosis and treatment of disease. The theory of Yin Yang and Five Elements has evolved into an important component part of TCM theory, and has exerted deep influence on the formation and development of the theoretical system of TCM.

Limited by the historic conditions, the materialistic and dialectical

11

ideas of the theory of Yin Yang and Five Elements in the ancient Chinese philosophy cannot be treated as the same with the materialistic dialectics in modern science.

Yin Yang Theory

Yin and Yang are a generalization of some related matter and phenomena, with opposite properties in nature. They stand for not only two opposite things, but also the two opposite aspects existing within one thing.

Yin Yang is a category of ancient Chinese philosophy. Its earliest meaning is facing or turning away from the sun. In other words, Yang refers to the side facing to the sun, while Yin refers to the side turning away from the sun. Afterwards, it is extended to mean the cold or hot of weather, upper or lower in locations, left or right, interior or exterior and motions or stillness. The ancient Chinese philosopher explained the two opposite forces of the nature which wane and wax alternately, believing that "all things contain Yin and Yang" and "Yin Yang serves as the law of nature".

According to Yin Yang theory, the material world is a unity resulting from the unity and opposite of Yin and Yang. Anything in the universe can be divided into the opposite Yin and Yang, such as the cold or hot of weather and the day and night. The contradictive movement of Yin and Yang lies in everything in the world, and occurrence, development and changes of all things in nature are the results of the contradictive movement of Yin and Yang in their opposing and supplementing.

It is necessary to know the following points in order to understand the concept of Yin and Yang: ① All the things or phenomena in the universe can be generalized as Yin and Yang. Generally speaking, things in violent movement, going outwards, ascending, warm, bright, etc. , belong to Yang; while those relatively still, hiding in the interior, going downwards, cold, dark, etc. , belong to Yin. As

12

for the human body, the substances and functions that can propel, warm and excite the human body belong to Yang; while those that can nourish the human body or cause stasis and inhibition of the human body, belong to Yang; ② The things summarized or divided by Yin Yang must be a pair of interrelated things or the two interrelated aspects of one thing, such as the heaven and earth, the sun and the moon, water and fire, and male and female; ③ The property of Yin and Yang of a thing is relative rather than absolute. This relativity, on the one hand, lies in that Yin and Yang may transform into each other in given condition, or, Yin can transform into Yang and vice versa. On the other hand, it lies in that things can be subdivided constantly, in other words, there is still Yin and Yang within a Yin thing or a Yang thing. For example, day belongs to Yang and night to Yin, but comparatively, morning belongs to Yang within the Yang and afternoon belongs to Yin within the Yang, and compared with the first part of the night, the later part of the night belongs to Yang within the Yin and the first part belongs to Yin within the Yin. Just as stated in *Yin Yang Li He Lun* (Treatise on Classification and Integration of Yin and Yang) in the book *Su Wen* (The Plain Questions): "Yin Yang can be used to classify the things limitlessly in accordance with the different levels of things, but the classifications must be all based on the basic properties of Yin and Yang. "

1. The basic contents of Yin Yang theory

(1) Mutual opposite and restriction between Yin and Yang: Yin Yang theory believes that Yin and Yang, the two opposite aspects, exist in all the things and phenomena in nature. The opposite of Yin and Yang indicates they have opposite properties, such as the opposite between motion and stillness, brightness and darkness, dryness and Dampness, and water and fire. The restriction of Yin and Yang refers to the two opposites existing in one unity, in continuous motion and change rather than stillness. As they are opposite in property, they restrict each other and repel each other, manifested as changes and movements of the thing. The process of the restriction between Yin and Yang is actually a process of wane and wax of Yin

and Yang. Without wane and wax of Yin and Yang, there will not be the restriction. Take cold and hot for example, the cold must restrict the hot, resulting in decline of the hot and growth of the cold and vice versa.

Yin and Yang are the unity of the opposite. The unity is the result of the opposite. The unity of the opposite Yin and Yang produces a dynamic equilibrium between them, which is known as coordination and balance of Yin and Yang. If this dynamic balance is disturbed, disaster in nature or disease in human body will follow. This is what is said in *Yin Yang Ying Xiang Da Lun* (Manifestations of Yin and Yang) in *Su Wen* (The Plain Questions) that "Excess of Yin will lead to disorder of Yang while Excess of Yang will cause disorder of Yin." Thus, the opposite and restriction between Yin and Yang serve as an important factor preventing Excess of either of Yin and Yang and maintaining their balance.

(2) Mutual dependence and supplement of Yin and Yang: This refers to that Yin and Yang, the opposites with opposite properties, depend on each other and supplement to each other, existing in one unity. Any of the Yin and Yang cannot exist without its opposite. For example, the upper belongs to Yang while the lower belongs to Yin. Without the upper, the lower can no longer be recongized, while without the lower, the upper never exists. The left belongs to Yang while the right belongs to Yin. Without the right, there is no left and vice verse, etc. As for the human body, the function is of Yang nature while the substance is of Yin nature. The substance exists within the body while the function is manifested in the exterior of the body. The substance existing in the interior provides basis for the generation of the functions, while the function manifested in the exterior is the manifestation of the substance in movement. The mutual dependence between Yin and Yang maintains the normal life activities. Either of them depends on its opposite for its existence. If the mutual dependence between Yin and Yang of the human body is destroyed due to some reasons, the normal life activities of the human body will be disturbed or even death may occur as a result of isolation of Yin and Yang.

14

The mutual dependence and supplement of Yin and Yang are a sign of the unity of the two opposites as well as a basis for the mutual transformation of Yin and Yang, because without the mutual dependence and supplement, the two opposite will not show the wane and wax and thus the transformation cannot occur.

(3) Wane and wax and balance between Yin and Yang: The balance through wane and wax between Yin and Yang indicates that the relative balance between Yin and Yang is maintained by the wane and wax between Yin and Yang. This balance is a dynamic process marked by wane of Yin and wax of Yang or vice versa that occurs in certain limit and period rather than a still or an absolute balance. For example, the weather changes gradually from cold to warm and further to hot from the winter to the spring and from the spring to the summer, which is a process in which the Yin declines and Yang grows; while it changes gradually from hot to cool and further to cold from the summer to the autumn and from the autumn to the winter, which is a process in which Yang declines and Yin grows. However, changes of cold and hot weather are about the same in one year, ensuing that the weather is kept in a balance. The restriction and dependence between Yin and Yang make the two opposites move and change constantly, thus the wane and wax of Yin and Yang are absolute while the balance is relative.

(4) Mutual transformation of Yin and Yang: This implies that the two opposite aspects of Yin and Yang may transform into each other under given conditions. In other words, Yin may transform into Yang and vice versa. It is a phenomenon that occurs when a thing goes to its extremity. If the wane and wax of Yin and Yang are regarded as a process of changes of things in quantity, transformation of Yin and Yang is in fact a change of quality developed from the change of quantity. For instance, the hottest point in summer that developed from the warm weather in spring is just the starting point for the weather to turn to cool or cold; while the coldest point in winter developed from the cool in autumn is just the starting point for the weather to turn to warm and hot. In the process of the development of disease, transformation of a Yang Syndrome into a Yin

one or vice versa is often encountered.

Both of the two opposite aspects have the intrinsic factors that cause the transformation. Besides, transformation between Yin and Yang depends on given conditions. Without the conditions, transformation is impossible.

In brief, Yin and Yang stand for the relative properties of things, which can be classified in accordance with Yin and Yang constantly. The mutual opposite and restriction of Yin and Yang, the mutual dependence and supplement, the wane and wax and balance as well as the transformation of Yin and Yang show that the relations between Yin and Yang are neither isolated nor still, instead they are interrelated and influenced, oppositing to each other and supplementing to each other. The mutual restriction and dependence of Yin and Yang signify that Yin and Yang, things or phenomena with different properties, exist in one unity; while the mutual restriction, supplement and transformation indicate that the opposite Yin and Yang are always in a state of movement and change caused by the restriction, supplement and transformation, and the wane and wax and ensuing the balance of Yin and Yang show that Yin and Yang maintain their relative dynamic balance in an absolute wane and wax movement.

2. Application of Yin Yang theory in TCM

Yin Yang theory penetrates through all aspects of TCM theory and is adopted to explain the structures, physiological functions, and law of occurrence and development of disease and to guide diagnosis and treatment of disease.

(1) Explaining the structures of the human body: TCM holds that the human body is an organic unity. According to the idea of the opposite of unity of Yin Yang theory, the opposites of unity of Yin Yang also exist in all aspects of the human body. The Zang Fu organs, meridians and other organs and tissues of the human body, on one hand, are closely related to each other, on the other, can be classified as two opposite aspects, Yin and Yang. Generally speaking, the upper of the human body pertains to Yang, while the lower to Yin; the exterior of the human body belongs to Yang, while the

16

interior to Yin. Compared with the trunk, the limbs belong to Yang while the trunk belongs to Yin; the back of the trunk belongs to Yang, while the abdomen to Yin, the lateral side of the limbs belongs to Yang, while the medial side to Yin. As for the Zang Fu organs, the Five Zang organs are located in the interior relatively and function to store essence instead of discharging food residues, so they belong to Yin; while the Six Fu organs, located in the exterior relatively and function to transform and transport foodstuff, belong to Yang. Of the Five Zang organs, the Heart and the Lung are situated in the upper part of the body (the thoracic cavity), so they belong to Yang; while the Spleen, the Liver and the Kidney, which are located in the lower (abdominal cavity), belong to Yin. As for each of the Zang Fu organs, it also includes Yin and Yang. For example, the Heart can be divided into the Heart Yin and the Heart Yang, the Kidney into the Kidney Yin and the Kidney Yang, etc. In a word, the opposites of Yin Yang unity are included in all the organs and tissues of the body, such as the upper and lower, the interior and exterior, the lateral side and medial side and the internal organs. Just as *Bao Ming Quan Xing Lun* (Treatise on Preserving Health) of the book *Su Wen* (The Plain Questions) states: "All the body structures can be classified in accordance with Yin and Yang."

(2) Expounding the physiological functions of the human body: Yin Yang theory is also used to explain the physiological functions of the human body, holding that the normal life activities arise from the coordination of Yin and Yang, or the opposites of the unity. For example, functions, compared with substance, belong to Yang while the substance to Yin. The relations between them are a concrete manifestation of relations between Yin and Yang. The physiological function of the human takes the substance as its material basis. Without the material basis such as the Zang Fu organs, meridians and Qi and Blood, there is no physiological functions, while the functions bring about constant metabolism of the substance. The relations between function and substance are just the relations of mutual dependence and mutual wane and wax between Yin and Yang. If Yin and Yang isolate from each other and fail to keep their mutual

supplementing effect, the human life will end. So, it is said in the *Sheng Qi Tong Tian Lun* (Communication of Qi of Man with Nature) in the book *Su Wen* (The Plain Questions): "When the relations between Yin and Yang in the body are kept normal, the body's functions as well as the body structure will be normal; while when the Yin and Yang of the body isolate from each other, life will end."

(3) Explaining the pathological changes of the human body: The cordinative Yin Yang relations should exist between the interior and exterior, the lateral and the medial, the upper and the lower, the different substances, the different functions, and the substance and the functions in order to maintain the normal physiological activities. If the coordination between Yin and Yang are disturbed due to certain reasons, diseases will occur as a result of Excess or Deficiency of Yin or Yang.

The occurrence and development of disease concern with both the Vital Qi and the pathogen. The Vital Qi indicates the structure and function of the human body as well as the resistant ability of the body against disease. The pathogen refers to various kinds of causative factors of disease. Properties of the Vital Qi and the pathogen and the process of their mutual action and struggle can all be explained by Yin and Yang or their movement and change. The process of a disease is just a process of struggle between the Vital Qi and the pathogen. Therefore, no matter how complicated a disease is in its occurrence, development and change, it can be summarized as Excess or Deficiency of Yin or Yang.

① Excess of Yin or Yang: This is a morbid state marked by either Yin or Yang exceeding its normal level.

Excess of Yang: This refers to the pathogenesis of a group of disease caused by invasion of a Yang pathogen and the combination of the Yang pathogen with Yang Qi of the human body, marked by absolute hyperactivity of Yang. Yang Excess will cause Heat and tend to impair Yin, because Yang stands for Heat and Yang restricts Yin. When the Yang is excessive, it will restrict and consume the Yin Fluid, leading to impairment of Yin.

18

Excess of Yin: This is the pathogenesis of a group of disease caused by invasion of Yin pathogen on the human body and the combination of the Yin pathogen with the Yin of the body, marked by absolute hyperactivity of Yin. As Yin stands for Cold and restricts Yang, Excess of Yin will cause Cold and consume and restrict Yang, leading to Deficiency of Yang Qi.

② Deficiency of Yin or Yang: This is a morbid state marked by either Yin or Yang being less than normal.

Deficiency of Yang: This is a general term for Yang insufficiency, which often causes Cold. According to the dynamic equilibrium of Yin and Yang, Deficiency of either Yin or Yang will cause the relative hyperactivity of its opposite. Failure of the deficient Yang to restrict Yin thus causes the Cold.

Yin Deficiency: This is a general term for depletion of Yin Fluid of the human body, which often leads to Heat. Inability of the deficient Yin to restrict Yang causes relative hyperactivity of Yang and the ensuing Heat.

Although the pathological changes of disease are rather complicated, they can all be summarized as disturbance of Yin and Yang, either Excess or Deficiency. Excess of Yang causing Heat, Excess of Yin causing Cold, Yang Deficiency causing Cold and Yin Deficiency causing Heat are often regarded as the general law of pathogenesis.

③ Mutual impairment of Yin and Yang: This includes two kinds, Yin Deficiency involving Yang and Yang Deficiency involving Yin. According to Yin Yang theory, Yin and Yang are mutually dependent. When either Yin or Yang Deficiency develops to certain degree, it will influence its opposite, leading to Deficiency of the opposite and the ensuing occurrence of Deficiency of both Yin and Yang. This kind of pathological change is known as mutual impairment of Yin and Yang.

When Yang Deficiency further develops, it may fail to generate Yin Fluid, leading to concurrence of the Deficiency of both Yin and Yang, which is known as Yang Deficiency involving Yin. When Yin Deficiency advances, it may fail to produce Yang Qi, causing Deficiency of both Yin and Yang, which is known as Yin Deficiency involving Yang. Obviously, Deficiency of both Yin and Yang are the common result of Yang Deficiency involving Yin and Yin Deficiency involving Yang. Deficiency of Yin and Yang doesn't mean that Yin and Yang are kept in balance at a lower level, it is a state with Yin Deficiency or Yang Deficiency as its main aspect.

④ Transformation of Yin and Yang: When disturbance of Yin and Yang becomes severe, Yin or Yang may transform into each other in given conditions. In other words, a Yang Syndrome may turn into a Yin Syndrome and vice versa; a Cold Syndrome may turn into a Heat Syndrome and vice versa.

(4) Guiding diagnosis of disease: As imbalance of Yin and Yang serves as the intrinsic cause of occurrence and development of disease, Yin Yang can be adopted to analyze and differentiate the clinical manifestations of disease, though they may be very complicated. For example, the data concerning disease gained through the four diagnostic methods (observing, smelling and auscultation, inquiring and palpation), including the colour, sound, symptoms and pulse conditions, must be differentiated with Yin and Yang so that the Yin or Yang property of the Syndrome can be identified. So, it is said in *Yin Yang Ying Xiang Da Lun* (Manifestations of Yin and Yang) in the book *Su Wen* (The Plain Questions): " A skilled doctor will use Yin and Yang to differentiate the colours and pulse conditions in diagnosis of disease. "

(5) Guiding prevention and treatment of disease:

① Guiding health preservation and prevention of disease: TCM puts a high value on the prevention of disease. Theories on health preservation and prevention of disease are both based on the Yin Yang theory. It is believed that changes of the human Yin and Yang must be coincident with those in the four seasons of a year so that the disease can be prevented and the life span prolonged.

② Guiding treatment of disease: The Yin Yang theory plays an important role in determining the therapeutic principle and summarizing the properties and actions of herbs. As disturbance of Yin and Yang is the basic cause of occurrence and development of disease, regulating the relations of Yin and Yang by reinforcing the Deficiency and eliminating the Excess to restore the relative balance of Yin and Yang forms the basic principle of treating disease. For Excess of Yin or Yang, which is the pathogenesis of Excess Syndrome, reducing the excessive Yin or Yang serves as the general principle when the opposite still shows no Deficiency. Yang Excess causes Excess Syndrome of Heat type, so cool or cold drugs should be adopted to restrict the hyperactive Yang, which is known as "using cold drugs to treat Heat Syndrome"; while Yin Excess causes Excess Syndrome of Cold type and thus warm or hot drugs should be selected to restrict the hyperactive Yin, which is known as "using Heat drugs to treat Cold Syndrome". As for Deficiency of Yin or Yang, reinforcing the Deficiency acts as the basic therapeutic principle. As the Heat Syndrome caused by failure of the deficient Yin to restrict Yang and the ensuing hyperactivity of Yang is deficient in nature, it shouldn't be treated with drugs of cold nature directly, instead, drugs nourishing Yin should be selected to restrict the hyperactive Yang. This kind of treatment is called "treating Yin in the case of Yang disease (of Deficiency type)" in *Huang Di Nei Jing* (The Yellow Emperor's Internal Classics). If a Yin Excess is caused by failure of the deficient Yang to restrict Yin, pungent and warm drugs which functions to dispel Yin Cold should be avoided, instead, the treatment should be aimed at supplementing Yang or tonifying the Fire to reduce the Cold of Deficiency type. This method is termed in *Huang Di Nei Jing* (The Yellow Emperor's Internal Classics) "treating Yang in the case of Yin disease (of Deficiency type)". Besides, as Yin and Yang are supplementary to each other, Zhang Jingyue of the Ming Dynasty advocated that "seeking Yang from nourishing Yin" and "seeking Yin from supplementing Yang", which should be stressed in the treatment of Deficiency of both Yin and Yang.

The properties and actions of drugs are dependent upon the nature, taste and ascending, descending, floating and sinking of drugs, which can all be generalized and explained with the Yin Yang theory. For example, drugs have four kinds of nature, cold, cool, warm and hot, of which cool and cold belong to Yin, and warm and hot belong to Yang. Of the five kinds of tastes of drugs, pungent and sweet belong to Yang, while sour, bitter and salty belong to Yin. The drugs functioning to ascend and floating belong to Yang, while those functioning to descend and sink belong to Yin.

Treatment of disease is carried out by determining a correct therapeutic principle in accordance with the Excess or Deficiency of Yin or Yang, followed by choosing proper drugs in light of the Yin Yang properties of drugs in order to regulate the imbalance of Yin and Yang caused by disease and cure the disease.

Five Elements Theory

The Five Elements refer to wood, fire, earth, metal and water and their movement. Theory of the Five Elements is a cosmos outlook and methodology using the properties of the Five Elements and their mutual generation, mutual restriction, encroachment and violation to understand the world, explain the natural phenomena and the law of movement and changes of the nature.

The basic ideas of the Five Elements theory lie in that the universe is composed of five kinds of most basic substances, wood, fire, earth, metal and water, which produce all the things in nature by mixing and combining with each other. Therefore, all the things in nature can be classified as the Five Elements, and the law of mutual generation and mutual restriction is a general law of interelations of all the things in nature.

In the process of its formation, the theoretical system of TCM was deeply influenced by the Five Elements theory, which, like Yin Yang theory, was gradually evolved into an inseparable component part of the unique TCM theory.

1. The basic contents of Five Elements theory in TCM

(1) Properties of Five Elements: This understanding comes from the knowledge to the five kinds of substances, or the wood, fire, earth, metal and water, in nature. It is generally believed that the classic generalization of the properties of the Five Elements is from *Hong Fan* (Great Category) of the book *Shang Shu* (Great Book),

22

in which it goes: the water has a property of moistening and going downwards; the wood has a property of being both flexing and extending, the fire has a property of flaring up, the earth has a property of generating and growing, and the metal has a property of changing and purifying.

① Property of wood: The wood has a property of flexing and extending, which originally means that the sticks of tree can both flex and extend, going upwards and outwards. Thus the property of wood is extended to mean growing, ascending, going upwards freely, etc.

② Property of Fire: The Fire has a property of flaring up, which originally means that the Fire is warm and goes upwards. Thus the property of Fire is extended to mean being warm, ascending and flaring.

③ Property of earth: The earth has a property of generating and growing, which originally means that the earth is where crops are planted and gathered in. Thus the property of earth is extended to mean generating, carrying and receiving all the things, and hence the saying that the earth carries the other four elements and that the earth is the mother of all things on earth.

④ Property of metal: The metal has a property of changing, which means originally that the metal tools can change things on will of the human beings. Thus the property of metal is extended to mean changing, purifying, descending and astringing.

⑤ Property of water: The water has a property of moistening and going downwards, which originally means that water flows downwards to moisten everything. Thus the property of water is extended to mean nourishing, coldness, going downwards and storing.

(2) Classification of things in accordance with the Five Elements: With the methods of analogy and abstract deduction, the ancient Chinese doctors summarized Zang Fu organs, limbs, orifices, various functions of the human body and the natural phenomena related to the human body in accordance with the Five Elements theory as five major systems. The table on next page is just such a summarization based on records in *Huang Di Nei Jing* (The Yellow Emperor's Internal Classics).

Classification of things in accordance with Fiver Elements

Nature							Human Body					
Five Seasons	Five Climates	Five Colours	Five Locations	Five Tastes	Five Changes	Five Elements	Five Zang	Five Fu	Five Orifices	Five Tissues	Five Secretions	Five Emotions
Spring	Wind	Blue	East	Sour	Generate	Wood	Liver	Gall-bladder	Eye	Tendon	Tear	Anger
Summer	Summer Heat	Red	South	Bitter	Grow	Fire	Heart	Small Intestine	Tongue	Vessel	Sweat	Joy
Long-Summer	Damp	Yellow	Middle	Sweet	Trans-form	Earth	Spleen	Stomach	Mouth	Muscle	Saliva	Anxiety
Autumn	Dry	White	West	Pungent	Harvest	Metal	Lung	Large Intestine	Nose	Skin	Nasal discharge	Sorrow
Winter	Cold	Black	North	Salty	Store	Water	Kidney	Bladder	Ear	Bone	Spittle	Terror

(3) Generation, restriction, encroachment and violation between Five Elements: The purpose of attribution of things to the Five Elements in Five Elements theory is to explain the law of the movement and change of the things in mutual connection and coordination with the relations of generation, restriction, encroachment and violation among the Five Elements. Of the four kinds of relations, generation and restriction are used to explain the normal relations of things, while the encroachment and the violation, the abnormal relations of things. ① Generation and restriction: These are two normal relations existing in the Five Elements.

Generation: Generation refers to the assisting, growing and promoting realtions existing among the Five Elements in order. The order of generation in Five Elements is: wood generating fire, fire generating earth, earth generating metal, metal generating water, and water generating wood. This relation comes one by one endlessly. In this relation, each of the Five Elements has two kinds of connection, being generated and generating other, which is also known as the relation of mother and son in *Nan Jing* (The Difficult Classics). The element generating is the mother, while the element being generated, the son. Take the earth for example, earth generates metal, so the earth is the mother of the metal and the metal, the son of the earth.

Restriction: This refers to the restricting and inhibiting effects existing in the Five Elements in order. The order of the restriction is: wood restricting earth, earth restricting water, water restricting fire, fire restricting metal, and metal restricting wood. This relation also comes one by one in sequence endlessly.

Normal movement of things maintained by generation and restriction: Relations among the Five Elements are in a mobile state in which the elements generate and restrict constantly. The generation and restriction are inseparable, existing concurrently in things. Without generation, nothing will generate and grow; while without restriction, the coordinative movement and change of things will not be kept. Thus, things can maintain their relative balance only when the actions of both the generation and restriction exist together in the things. This is just what is said in *Liu Wei Zhi Da Lun* (A Great Treatise on Six Kinds of Secrets) in *Su Wen* (The Plain Questions): "Hyperactivity of the Five Elements will cause disaster, while coordination of generation and restriction is an imperative factor for normal development of things."

② Encroachment and violation: This is the abnormal restriction occurring when the normal relations of generation and restriction are destroyed.

Encroachment: Any of the Five Elements, if being excessive, will overrestrict the element it restricts, leading to destruction of the coordination and balance among the Five Elements. The order of encroachment is just the order of the restriction, or the wood encroaching earth, earth encroaching water, water encroaching fire, fire encroaching metal, and metal encroaching wood. There are two kinds of causes contributing to the encroachment: one is that one of the elements is too strong, so it exerts more stronger restriction on the element it restricts, which is comparatively deficient in this case; the other is that one of the elements is too weak to bear the normal restriction, so it often becomes even weaker. The former case is the encroachment due to Excess, while the latter is the encroachment due to Deficiency.

Violation: This refers to the counter restriction of one element on the element restricting it due to its hyperactivity. It is also a manifestation of disturbance of the normal relations among the Five Elements. Order of violation is thus just opposite to that of restriction: wood violating metal, metal violating fire, fire violating water, water violating earth, and earth violating wood. There are also two possibilities to cause violation: one is that one of the elements is so strong that it counterrestricts the element originally restricting it; the other is that one of the element is too weak to restrict the element it should restrict, instead it is restricted by the element.

Although the orders of encroachment and violation are opposite, they both are the abnormal signs of disturbance of the normal relations in the Five Elements. Therefore, they may occur concurrently.

26

2. Application of Five Elements theory in TCM

The Five Elements theory is so widely applied in TCM that it is used to not only explain the TCM theories but also to guide clinical practice.

(1) Explaining the physiological functions of the Five Zang organs and their relations: In the Five Elements theory, the Five Zang organs are ascribed to the Five Elements and thus the physiological functions of the Five Zang organs can be explained with the properties of the Five Elements.

Wood has the property of growing, going upwards freely and smoothly, the Liver Qi likes flowing freely and is averse to be stagnated, and the Liver functions to disperse, so the Liver is ascribed to wood; fire has the property of warming and flaring up, and the Heart can warm the body, so the Heart is ascribed to fire; the earth has the property of generating everything, and the Spleen dominates transformation and transportation of foodstuff and serves as the source of generation of Qi and Blood, so the Spleen is ascribed to the earth; the metal has the property of purifying and estranging, and the Lung Qi takes downward movement and purifying as its main features, so the Lung is ascribed to the metal; and the water has the property of moistening, being cold and going downwards, while the Kidney stores essence and dominates water metabolism, so the Kidney is ascribed to water.

In the Five Elements theory, the body structure including the Zang Fu organs and tissues are classified as the Five Elements and the natural phenomena such as the five regions, five seasons, five climatic conditions, five tastes and five colours are also categorized as the Five Elements, so the man and nature are unified in the Five Elements, showing that man is correspondent to the nature.

It should be pointed out that the explanation of the functions of the Five Zang organs with the Five Elements theory is carried out based on abstract deduction and analogy. It is incomplete in illustrating the functional activities of the Five Zang organs.

(2) Explaining the relations among the Five Zang organs: There are close interrelations among the functional activities of the Five

Zang organs, which can be explained with the generating and restricting effects among the Five Elements.

① Generating effect among the Five Zang organs: Ascribed to the Five Elements, the Five Zang organs also possess the relation of generation among the Five Elements. For example, the Liver, belonging to wood, can store Blood to assist the Heart Blood; the Yang Heat of the Heart which belongs to fire can warm the Spleen; the Spleen, belonging to earth, produces food essence to nourish the Lung; the Lung, belonging to metal, functions downwards to nourish the Kidney; and the Kidney, belonging to water, stores essence to aid in the Liver.

② Restricting effect among the Five Zang organs: The restricting relations in the Five Elements can be adopted to explain the restricting effects in the Five Zang organs. For example, the Liver belongs to wood, its dispersive effect can inhibit the stagnating property of the Spleen (earth); the Spleen belongs to earth, its transforming and transporting effect can prevent the Kidney water from overflowing; the Kidney belongs to water, ascending of its water can restrict the hyperactivity of the Heart Fire; the Heart belongs to fire, its warming effect can prevent the Lung Qi from descending too much; and the Lung belongs to metal, its descending and purifying effect can prevent the Liver Yang from rising excessively.

It is because of the mutual generation and mutual restriction among the Five Zang organs that the relative balance of the human body and the ensuing normal life activities are maintained.

(3) Explaining influence of diseases of the Five Zang organs: Being closely related with each other in physiology, the Five Zang organs certainly influence each other in pathology. Disease of a Zang organ may be transmitted to another organ or transformed from another organ. This kind of influence in pathology is known as transmission of disease, which can be divided into two different conditions when explained with the Five Elements theory.

① Transmissions in accordance with the generating effect: This include disease of a mother organs affecting the son organ and that of the son organ affecting the mother.

Disease of the mother organ affecting the son organ: This is a transmission of disease from the mother organ to the son organ. For example, the Kidney belongs to water and the Liver belongs to wood, so the Kidney is the mother organ while the wood is the son organ. If disease of the Kidney affects the Liver, it will be an example of disease transmitting from the mother organ to the son organ. Insufficiency of the essence and Blood of the Liver and Kidney and failure of the water to nourish the wood, which are commonly seen in clinic, are just such examples.

Disease of the son organ affecting the mother organ: This is also called the son depriving the mother Qi, referring to a disease transmitting from the son organ to the mother organ. For example, the Liver belongs to wood, and the Heart belongs to fire, so the Liver is the mother of the Heart and the Heart is the son of the Liver. If disease of the Heart affects the Liver, it will be an example of the disease transmitting from the son to the mother. Blood Deficiency of both the Heart and the Liver and hyperactivity of Fire of both the Heart and the Liver are just such examples commonly seen in clinic.

② Transmission in accordance with the restricting effect: This include two aspects: transmission of disease according to the encroachment of the Five Elements and that according to the violation of the Five Elements.

Transmission of disease according to the encroachment: This refers to transmission of disease of one organ to the organ it restricts originally. The laws of the transmission are, disease of Liver transmitting to the Spleen, that of the Spleen to the Kidney, that of the Kidney to the Heart, that of the Heart to the Lung, and that of the Lung to the Liver. Such Syndromes as transverse attack of the Liver Qi on the Stomach or the Spleen are just such examples commonly seen in clinic.

Transmission of disease according to the violation: This refers to transmission of disease of an organ to the organ restricting it originally. The laws of transmission are: disease of the Liver transmitting to the Lung, that of the Lung to the Heart, that of the Heart to the Kidney, that of the Kidney to the Spleen, and that of the Spleen to the Liver. Such Syndromes as attack of the Liver Qi or the Liver Fire on the Lung are just such examples.

In the view of the Five Elements theory, all the transmission of disease among the Five Zang organs can be explained with the generation, restriction, encroachment and violation of the Five Elements. When disease transmits according to the law of generation, disease from the mother organ to the son organ is relatively mild; while disease from the son to the mother is severe. When disease transmits according to restriction, disease transmitting in light of encroachment is severe, while that in light of the violation is mild.

It should be pointed out that the coordinative connections among the Five Zang organs mainly depend on the mutual influence and mutual actions of their physiological functions, so they cannot be completely elaborated with the generating and restricting effects among the Five Elements. Therefore, transmission of disease among the Five Zang organs, in the same way, does not always follow the laws of the orders of generation, restriction, encroachment and violation in the Five Elements.

(4) Guiding diagnosis and treatment:

① Guiding diagnosis of disease: Man is an organic unity. Disease of the internal organs with corresponding abnormal changes of their functional activities and disturbance of their connections may be reflected on the tissues and organs on the exterior of the human body, manifested as abnormal changes of the colour, lustre, voice, shape and pulse condition. Since the Five Zang organs, five colours, five sounds and five tastes are all ascribed to the Five Elements, diagnosis of disease can be performed by generalizing the data gained through observing, smelling and auscultation, inquiring and palpating by the aid of the law of transmission of disease in accordance with the generation, restriction, encroachment and violation among the Five Elements. For instance, a Liver disease may be diagnosed when a patient presents a greenish face, inclination to eat sour food and a wiry pulse. If a patient originally with Heart disease marked by stuffiness in the precordial region exhibits a dark face and inability to lie flat, he or she may be diagnosed as having attack of the

30

Kidney water on the Heart.

② Guiding treatment: Controlling transmission of disease: Disease may transform from one organ to another and vice versa. So treatment should be directed not only at the diseased organ, but also at the regulation of relations among the Five Zang organs in accordance with generation, restriction, encroachment and violation of the Five Elements. To be more exact, excessive Syndrome should be treated with reducing method, and Deficiency Syndrome by reinforcing method, with a view to controlling the transmission of disease. For example, Liver disease may affect the Heart, the Spleen, the Lung and the Kidney in accordance with the laws of generation, restriction, encroachment and violation in Five Elements, or it may be the result of transmission of disease from the Heart, the Spleen, the Lung and the Kidney. In the case of hyperactive Liver Qi, strengthening the Spleen and Stomach should be adopted to prevent the disease transmitting from the Liver to the Spleen and Stomach, as hyperactive wood will overrestrict the earth. If the Spleen and Stomach is strengthened, disease will not transmit and is relatively easy to cure. For this reason, it is pointed out in *Nan Jing* (The Difficult Classics) that "One should know that Liver disease would transmit to the Spleen and thus strengthening the Spleen should be done first."

In clinic, doctor should master the relations of generation, restriction, enchroachment and violation of the Five Elements in order to control the transmission of disease. What is more, he should give treatment in accordance with the Syndromes identified instead of adhering to the law of the disease transmission based on the relations of the Five Elements rigidly.

Determining therapeutic principle and method: Many therapeutic principles and methods can be made based on the Five Elements theory, the following of which are commonly used in clinic.

Therapeutic principles determined in the law of the generation relation of the Five Elements: When disease is treated with the generation relations of the Five Elements, the basic principles are tonifying the mother in the case of Deficiency and reducing the son in the

31

case of Excess.

Tonifying mother is mainly adopted to treat the Deficiency Syndrome concerning the mother-son relationship. For example, Syndrome of water failing to nourish wood marked by Deficiency of the Liver Yin due to the deficient Kidney Yin being unable to nourish the Liver should be treated by nourishing the Kidney instead of nourishing the Liver directly. This is because the Kidney is the mother of the Liver, so nourishing the Kidney can promote the Liver, which is known as tonifying the mother causing restoration of the son.

Reducing the son is mainly used to treat Excess Syndrome concerning the mother and the son. For example, Excess Syndrome of the Liver caused by hyperactivity of the Liver Fire may be treated by purging the Heart Fire. This is because the Liver is the mother of the Heart and purging the Heart Fire can help to reduce the Liver Fire.

Clinically, even a disease involving only one organ may also be treated according to the principle tonifying the mother and reducing the son.

Therapeutic methods made in the law of the generating relation of the Five Elements: The ones commonly used are as follows:

Nourishing water to restrict wood: This is a method of supplementing the Liver Yin by nourishing the Kidney, suitable for treatment of hyperactivity of Liver Yang due to Deficiency of both the Liver Yin and the Kidney Yin.

Supplementing the fire to strengthen the earth: This is a method of supplementing the Spleen Yang by warming up the Kidney Yang, used to treat Syndrome of Deficiency of the Spleen Yang caused by Kidney Yang Deficiency. According to the generation and restriction in the Five Elements, the Heart belongs to fire and the Spleen belongs to earth, so failure of fire to generate earth should indicate failure of the Heart Fire to generate the Spleen earth. However, since upsurging of the Mingmen theory, the meaning of failure of fire to generate earth has extended to mean the Syndrome of Deficiency of both the Kidney Yang and the Spleen Yang due to failure of the Mingmen Fire or the Kidney Yang to warm the Spleen Yang, rarely meaning the relations between the Heart Fire and the Spleen Yang.

Building up the earth to generate metal: This is a method of supplementing the Spleen Qi to generate the Lung Qi, used to treat Deficiency of the Spleen and Stomach failing to nourish the Lung and the ensuing Deficiency of both the Spleen and the Lung.

Generating both the water and the metal: This is a method of tonifying both the Lung Yin and the Kidney Yin, which is marked by treating these two organs at the same time. It is suitable for Deficiency of both the Lung Yin and the Kidney Yin caused by either failure of the deficient Lung to distribute Body Fluid to nourish the Kidney or by failure of the deficient Kidney Yin to send up essence to the Lung.

The therapeutic principles and methods determined in the law of the restricting relations of the Five Elements:

Therapeutic principles made n the law of the restricting relations of the Five Elements: Although pathological changes in the clinic may be divided into over-restriction, inadequate restriction and counter restriction in accordance with the Five Elements theory, they can be generalized as two aspects, being too strong or being too weak. The "strong" refers to the element restricting in pathological conditions, which is marked by hyperactivity of the functional activity; while the "weak" refers to the elements being restricted which is characterized by decline of the functional activity. Therefore, the therapeutic principles made based on the restricting relations of the Five Elements are mainly twofold, reducing the strong and reinforcing the weak, and in most cases, they are adopted in combination with reducing the strong as the main aspect to help the weak to restore.

Reducing the strong may be used to treat Syndrome marked by over-restriction. For example, the Syndrome of hyperactive Liver attacking the earth marked by the transverse attack of the Liver Qi on the Stomach and the Spleen should be treated by soothing the flow of the Liver Qi and suppressing the Liver. If accumulation of

Damp Heat or Damp Cold obstructs free flow of the Liver Qi and causes earth violating wood, the treatment should be aimed at promoting transformation and transportation of the Spleen and regulating the function of the Stomach.

Reinforcing the weak may be used to treat inadequate restriction. For example, the Syndrome of failure of the Liver to dredge the earth marked by the deficient Liver Qi leading to disturbance of the transforming and transporting effects of the Spleen should be mainly treated by regulating the Liver Qi and supported by strengthening the Spleen.

Therapeutic methods made in the law of the restricting relation of the Five Elements: The commonly adopted are as follows:

Suppressing the wood to support the earth: This is a method of treating hyperactivity of Liver and Deficiency of Spleen by soothing flow of the Liver Qi and strengthening the Spleen, which is also known as the method of soothing flow of Liver Qi and strengthening the Spleen, suppressing the Liver to regulate the function of the Stomach, or regulating functions of both the Liver and the Spleen. It is suitable for treating encroachment of the hyperactive wood on the earth or failure of the wood to dredge the earth.

Supplementing the earth to restrict water: This is a method of treating retention of water by warming up the Spleen Yang or warming up the Kidney Yang and strengthening the Spleen, used to treat edema and abdominal fullness and distention caused by failure of the Spleen to perform its transforming and transporting effect and the resultant overflow of water. In the case of retention of water due to inability of the Kidney to perform its effect in controlling water metabolism and failure of the Spleen to transform and transport water as a result of the deficient Kidney Yang being unable to warm the Spleen Yang, it is a case of counter restriction of the water on the earth and should be treated mainly by warming up the Kidney Yang by the aid of supporting the Spleen Yang.

Assisting the metal to suppress the wood: This is a method marked by assisting the descending and purifying effects of the Lung to suppress the Liver, which is also known as purging the Liver and

34

clearing the Lung, used mostly to treat hyperactivity of the Liver Fire leading to failure of the Lung Qi to descend.

Purging the south and supplementing the north: This refers to purging the Heart Fire and nourishing the Kidney water, also known as purging fire and tonifying water or nourishing Yin and reducing Fire. It is often adopted to treat incoordination between the Heart and Kidney marked by the deficient Kidney Yin failing to nourish the Heart Yin and the ensuing hyperactivity of the Heart Fire. It is so named because the Heart dominates fire which corresponds to the south and the Kidney dominates water which corresponds to the north.

In TCM, the Five Elements theory not only guides treatment with drugs, but also guides the treatment with acupuncture, moxibustion and psychological therapy.

The Yin Yang theory and the Five Elements theory both have their own characteristics, but they have close relations and in fact they are applied in combination in medical field. Both of them take their own properties and the relations among them as the theoretical guidance, and the physiological and pathological manifestations as the objective basis in analysis and illustration of the physiological functions and pathological changes of the human body. Therefore it is necessary to combine these two theories with each other when analyzing and treating disease in the clinic.

The life activities of the human body and the relations between man and nature are very complicated, and the Yin Yang and the Five Elements theories are far from accomplishment as a result of the limitation of the historic and social conditions. Therefore, one shouldn't limit his study on the abstract philosophical concepts of Yin Yang or Five Elements while researching the life activities of the human body, including both the physiological functions and the pathological changes.

Viscera-state
Theory

*I*n TCM, viscera-state theory is also known as Zang Xiang theory. Zang refers to the visceras in the interior of the body, while Xiang refers to the outwards manifestations of the visceral organs.

The viscera-state theory is a subject dealing with the physiological functions and pathological changes of Zang Fu organs and the relations among the Zang Fu organs. It is an important component part of TCM theory. This theory mainly includes three contents: the morphology and physiological functions of the Zang Fu organs; the relations between the Five Zang organs, the limbs, the orifices and the secretions; and the relations among the Zang Fu organs.

The viscera-state theory takes Zang Fu as its basis, which is a general term for all the internal organs. According to the features of their different physiological functions, Zang Fu can be classified as three groups, Zang organs, Fu organs and the extraordinary Fu organs. There are Five Zang organs, namely, the Heart, the Lung, the Spleen, the Liver and the Kidney, which are collectively called the Five Zang organs. Six Fu organs consist of the Stomach, the Gallbladder, the Large Intestine, the Small Intestine, the Bladder and the Triple Jiao, known collectively as the Six Fu organs, and the extraordinary organs include the brain, marrow, bone, vessel, Bladder and the uterus. The common physiological features of the Five Zang organs are to store and generate essence, while those of the Six Fu organs, to receive, transform and transport foodstuff. The extraordinary organs differ from the Six Fu organs in physiological functions and shape. They don't contact with foodstuff, are relatively sealed organs and can store essence Qi as the Five Zang organs. Thus it is stated in *Wu Zang Bie Lun* (Supplementary Discussion on Five Zang Organs) in *Su Wen* (The Plain Questions): "The Five Zang organs function to store essence instead of discharging food residues, so they allow the essence Qi rather than the foodstuff to fill with them, while the Six Fu organs function to transform and transport foodstuff, so they allow foodstuff instead of the essence Qi to fill with them."

The viscera-state theory has evolved into a relatively complete system by the time of *Huang Di Nei Jing* (The Yellow Emperor's Internal Classics). Its formation is mainly based on three points: the anatomical knowledge of the ancient Chinese, long-standing observation on the physiological functions and pathological changes of the human body, and the accumulation and summarization of long-term clinical practice. Doctors of the later generations, under the guidance of the traditional theory, enriched and developed the viscera-state theory gradually through their own clinical observation and practice. Up to today, this theory still serves as the most important theoretical basis for clinical practice.

Concept of wholism with the Five Zang organs as its core is the most basic feature of the viscera-state theory. This is mainly manifested by: Zang and Fu organs being interior-exteriorly related, interrelations between the Five Zang organs and the orifices and body tissues of the body, and close relations between the physiological functions of the Five Zang organs with the spirit and emotional states. In other words, the body is integrated into a unity with the Five Zang organs as the core by ascribing the other organs and orifices of the body as well as the spirit, mental activities and emotional states to the Five Zang organs, with a view to explain the integrity and unity of the body's internal environment with the promoting and restricting relations among the Five Zang organs. Meanwhile, the physiological functions adjust themselves alongside the changes of the natural environment, from which the coordination and balance between man and nature are maintained. The connections between the Five Zang organs and the orifices, spirit and mental activities are the way for the internal and external environments of the human body to communicate, which maintains the coordination and balance of internal and external environments of the human body.

Although the concept of wholism in viscera-state theory takes the ancient anatomical knowledge as a part of its basis, its formation and development are mainly realized by adopting such researching methods as knowing the interior by analyzing the exterior and the analogy methods based on Yin Yang and Five Elements theory. Therefore, knowledge of the Zang Fu organs gained through such observating and analyzing methods are much more than that gained only through the anatomical visceral organs of the human body, thus forming the unique theoretical system of physiology and pathology of TCM. For this reason, although such Zang Fu organs as the Heart, the Lung, the spleen, the Liver and the Kidney in viscera-state theory share the same names with those in Western medicine, they are somewhat different in their physiological functions and pathological changes. The functional activities of one organ in the viscera-state theory of TCM may inlude the physiological functions of several organs in Western medicine, while the physiological functions of a visceral organ in Western medicine, may concern with those of several organs in the viscera-state theory. To be more exact, the Zang Fu organs in the viscera-state theory is a physiological and pathological concept involving a system of the human body, including the anatomical visceral organs.

The Five Zang Organs

The Five Zang organs refers to the Heart, the Lung, the Spleen, the Liver and the Kidney. In meridian theory, sometimes the pericardium is also regarded as one Zang organ, so there is the saying of six Zang organs. The Five Zang organs have different physiological functions, but the functional activities of the Heart play a leading role. Such relations as mutual dependence, mutual restriction and mutual coordination among the Five Zang organs are explained in TCM based on Yin Yang and Five Elements theory, and the physiological functions of the Five Zang organs are closely related to the changes of the natural environment and the emotional states.

1. The Heart

The Heart is located in the thorax between the two Lungs about the diaphragm, like an upside down lotus in shape, and surrounded by the pericardium. It is where the spirit is housed and controls Blood and vessels. In Five Elements theory, it is ascribed to fire and thus governs the life activities. So, it is called the monarch organ in *Ling Lan Mi Dian Lun* (Extremely Important Treatise) in *Su Wen* (The Plain Questions). The main functions of the Heart are to dominate Blood and Blood vessels and controls mental activity. Besides, it opens into the tongue, has its specific manifestations on the face, and is related to joy in emotions and sweat in secretions. Because of the mutual pertaining and connecting of the meridians, the Heart has an interior-exterior relationship with the Small Intestine.

(1) Main functions of the Heart:

① Controlling Blood and Blood vessels: This includes two points, the Heart controlling Blood and dominating vessels. All the Blood of the body depends on the propelling of the Heart for their flowing in the vessels and thus Blood can be sent to the whole body to nourish the body. Vessels, also known as meridians, are where Blood circulates, so flow of Blood is also influenced by whether the vessels are smooth or not.

39

It is the Heart Qi that maintains the normal Heart beats and the normal circulation of Blood in the vessels. When the Heart Qi is sufficient, there is normal heart force, heart rate and heart rhythm, and the normal circulation of Blood in the vessels. As a result of sufficient supply of Blood, the face is red and lustrous and the pulse is felt moderate and forceful. Moreover, the functional state of the Heart Qi is also related to the vicissitude of the pectoral Qi.

The normal circulation of Blood also depends on adequate filling of Blood in the vessels. In the case of Blood Deficiency, the vessels will be less filled and the normal Heart beats and the flow of Blood will be disturbed. So, normal flow of Blood is determined by sufficient Heart Qi, adequate filling of vessels and smoothness of the vessels. If there is Heart Qi Deficiency, Blood Deficiency or obstruction of the vessels, Blood will flow sluggishly or the vessels will become insufficiently filled, leading to such manifestations as lustreless face and fine and weak pulse, or even to stagnation of Qi and Blood Stasis due to obstruction of vessels which is marked by dim and greyish face, purplish tongue and lips, stuffiness and stabbing pain in the precardial region and knotted, intermittent, running or uneven pulse. From this we can see that the so-called Heart dominating Blood and Blood vessels indicates the physiological functions of the relatively independent system formed by the Heart, Blood and vessels. Disturbance of any of the three will cause disturbance of the function of the Heart in dominating Blood or Blood vessels.

② Controlling mental activity: This is also known as the spirit being housed in the Heart. *Shen* in Chinese has two meanings. In a broad sense, it refers to the outward manifestations of the life activities, such as the body forms, complexion, eyesight, speech and the postures of limbs; while in a narrow sense, it indicates the spirit dominated by the Heart, or the spirit, consciousness and mental activities.

According to Western medicine, the spirit, thinking and consciousness, as the responses of the brain to the external events, are the functional activities of the brain. But in the viscera-state theory which takes the Five Zang organs as its center, the spirit, thinking and consciousness are ascribed to the Five Zang organs and the Heart is regarded as the "king" of all the organs of the body, so it is the Heart instead of the brain that dominates mental activities. It is clearly pointed out in *Ling Lan Mi Dian Lun* in *Su Wen* (The Plain Questions) that "The Heart is a monarch organ which controls the mental activities." When the Heart governs the mental activities normally, there will be a vigorous spirit, clear mind, quick thinking and quick response to the external stimuli. If the Heart fails to control the mental activities, disturbance of the spirit, consciousness and thinking will occur, manifested as insomnia, dream-disturbed sleep, restlessness or even delirium, or manifested as slow response, forgetfulness, listlessness or even coma.

The function of the Heart in controlling mental activities is closely related to the function of the Heart in controlling Blood and vessels. Blood is the material basis of spirit. It is just because the Heart controls Blood and vessels that it has the function of controlling the mental activities. This is why there will always be abnormal changes of the mental activities when the function of the Heart is disturbed.

(2) Connection between the Heart and the emotions, secretions, body tissues and orifices:

① Related to joy in emotions: In the viscera-state theory, the five kinds of emotional state, or joy, anger, anxiety, sorrow (worry) and terror, have close relationships with the functional states of the Five Zang organs. That the Heart is related to joy means that the physiological functions of the Heart is closely related to the joy, which is a favorable response of the human body to the external stimuli and thus is beneficial to such physiological functions of the Heart as controlling Blood and vessels and to both the body and mind. However, overjoy may damage the Heart spirit and causes the Heart Qi to disperse. Or the other way round, if the function of the Heart in controlling spirit is too strong, persistent laugh may appear; while liability to become sorrow is likely to occur when this function is inadequate.

② Related to sweat in secretions: Sweat is the liquid discharged from the sweat pore, which is produced by the steaming effect of

Yang Qi on the Body Fluid. As the sweat comes from the Body Fluid and both the Body Fluid and Blood controlled by the Heart are produced by food essence, it is said that the Heart is related to sweat in secretions and that the sweat and Blood have common source. Therefore, profuse sweating may impair the Yang Qi of the Heart, leading to palpitation, shortness of breath, listlessness or even coma with cold limbs. Besides, Deficiency of the Heart Qi or the Heart Yin may cause spontaneous sweating or night sweating.

③ Related to vessels in body tissues and having its specific manifestations on the face: That the Heart is related to vessels means all the vessels of the body are controlled by the Heart, and that the Heart has its specific manifestations on the face means that the functional states of the Heart can be reflected as the changes of the colour and luster of the face. As the face and head are extremely rich in Blood vessels, sufficiency of the Heart Qi and filling of vessels with enough Blood will be manifested as a red and lustrous face, while deficiency of the Heart Qi will cause the face to be puffy and pale or dark, Deficiency of Heart Blood will cause a lustreless face, and obstruction of the Heart vessels will cause a purplish face.

④ Opening into the tongue: The main functions of the tongue are to taste and assist speak. That the Heart opens into the tongue means that we can learn the functional states of the Heart in controlling Blood and spirit from the condition of the tongue. If the Heart functions properly, the tongue will be red, moist, soft and flexible in movement, with a quick tasting and fluent speech. If the Heart Qi is deficient, the tongue will be pale and tender. If the Heart Yin is deficient, the tongue will be red or deep red and emaciated. If the Heart Fire flares up, the tongue will be red or even exhibit erosions or ulcers. If the Heart vessel is blocked, the tongue will be dim, purplish or with acchymosis. If the Heart fails to control mental activities, the tongue will be curved and rigid, with aphasia or difficult speech. Therefore, there is the saying that the tongue is the outward manifestation of the Heart or that the tongue is the sprout of the Heart.

2. The Lung

The Lungs are located in the thoracic cavity, each of which is on either side. Among the Zang Fu organs, the Lung is in the uppermost, so it is described as a "carriage roof". As the Lung is intolerable to both cold and heat and tends to be attacked by pathogens due to its tender lobes, it is also known as tender organ in TCM. This organ belongs to metal in Five Elements and its main functions are to dominate Qi and respiration, tend to go outwards and downwards, regulate water metabolism, meet with all the vessels of the body and assist the Heart to govern the whole body by regulating flow of Qi and Blood. It communicates with the throat in its upper part and is related to skin and hairs in tissues, sorrow in emotions and nasal discharge in secretions, and opens into the nose. As both of the Lung Channel of Hand-Taiyin and the Large Intestinal Channel of Hand-Yangming connect with or pertain to the Lung and Large Intestine respectively, the Lung and the Large Intestine have an interior-exterior relationship.

(1) The main functions of the Lung:

① Dominating Qi and respiration: Qi dominated by the Lung includes both the Qi of the whole body and that of respiration. That the Lung dominates Qi of respiration means that the Lung dominates respiration, which is one of the functional activities of the Lung in dominating Qi. It is specially suggested here because it is very important.

Dominating Qi of the whole body: This means that all the Qi of the whole body is controlled by the Lung. This is mainly manifested as two points: firstly, the Lung Qi communicates with the heaven Qi. Qi of the human body, especially the pectorial Qi, depends on combination of the food essence transformed by the Spleen and the Stomach and the fresh air inhaled by the Lung for its formation, therefore functional states of the Lung influences the formation of the pectoral Qi and the Qi of the whole body. Secondly, the Lung has a regulating effect on the movement of Qi of the whole body, because the Lungs' respiration is one kind of ascending, descending, outgoing and entering movements of Qi, and its rhythmic movement contributes greatly to the maintenance and regulation of the movement of Qi of the whole body.

Dominating Qi of respiration: This indicates that the Lung has the respiratory effect. The Lung is where the fresh air in the nature and the turbid Qi of the body exchanges. Through the respiration of the Lung, the fresh air in the sky is inhaled and the turbid Qi of the body is exhaled, to ensure the normal change of gases. The continuous exhalation of the turbid Qi and the inhalation of the fresh air promote the formation of Qi and regulate the ascending, descending, outgoing and entering movement of Qi so that the human metabolism can be carried out normally. The respiratory effect of the Lung plays an extremely important role in the life activities. An even and normal respiration is the prerequisite for the smooth flow of Qi in the body, and it is just because the Lung dominates respiration that the Lung has the effect of dominating Qi of the whole body. If the respiratory effect of the Lung is disturbed, it will certainly influence the formation of the pectoral Qi and the movement of Qi, leading to weakening of the Lung in dominating Qi. If the Lung loses its respiratory effect, with the fresh air failing to be inhaled and the turbid Qi failing to be exhaled, the life activities of the human body will end. In the same way, Deficiency of Qi and disturbance of Qi's movement as well as abnormal distribution and discharge of Blood and Body Fluid may disturb the respiratory effect of the Lung, leading to abnormal respiration.

② Dominating dispersing and descending: That the Lung dominates dispersing indicates that the Lung Qi has a tendency of going upwards and outwards, while that the Lung dominates descending means that the Lung Qi tends to go downwards and has the effect of keeping the respiration clean.

Dominating dispersing: This is mainly manifested as three aspects: firstly, the Lung sends out the turbid Qi of the whole body by the dispersing effect; secondly, the Lung sends the Body Fluid and the food essence transported by the Spleen to the whole body, especially the superficial; and thirdly, it sends the defensive Qi outward to the skin so that the defensive Qi can regulate the opening-closing movement of the sweat pores and the metabolized Body Fluid

44

can be turned into sweat to be discharged. Therefore, failure of the Lung Qi to perform its dispersive effect often leads to difficult exhalation, chest distention, cough, asthma, nasal obstruction, sneeze and absence of sweating.

Dominating descending: As the Lung is in the uppermost among Zang Fu organs, the Lung Qi tends to go downwards. This effect is also mainly manifested as three aspects: firstly, it can inhale the fresh air in nature and send it down to the Kidney to be received by the Kidney; secondly, it can send the fresh air inhaled by the Lung, the Body Fluid and the food essence transported by the Spleen downwards; and thirdly, it can clean the foreign bodies in the respiratory tract and the Lung to keep the respiratory tract clean. Therefore, when the Lung Qi fails to descend, it may cause shortness of breath or shallowness of breath, cough with sputum, or hemoptysis.

The dispersing effect and the descending effect of the Lung are both opposite to each other and supplementary to each other. Under physiological conditions, they depend on each other and restrict each other, while under pathological conditions, they influence each other. If the Lung can perform its dispersing and descending effects normally, the respiratory tract will be smooth, the respiration will be even and the gas inside and outside the body can be exchanged. If their relations are disturbed, there will be failure of the Lung Qi to disperse or failure of the Lung Qi to descend, manifested as dyspnea, cough, upward attack of the Lung Qi, etc.

③ Regulating metabolism of water: This refers to that the Lung has the function of dredging and regulating the distribution and discharge of water through its dispersing and descending effects. The dispersing effect of the Lung can not only send the Body Fluid and food essence to the whole body, but also can control the opening and closing of the striae of muscles to adjust discharge of sweat; while the descending effect of the Lung can not only send downwards the fresh air to the Kidney, but also can send downwards the water of the body, the surplus water of which is then turned into urine to be discharged under the action of the steaming effect of the Kidney and

45

Bladder. Therefore, the Lung plays an important role in regulating water metabolism, and hence the saying that the Lung dominating distribution of water and the Lung being the upper source of water. When this effect is weakened, water will retain in the body, leading to Phlegm or water retention, or even edema as a result of overflow of water.

④ Meeting with all the Blood vessels and assisting the Heart to govern the whole body: All the Blood of the body meets in the Lung where it performs exchange of air and then is sent to the whole body again through the respiration of the Lung. Blood and vessels of the whole body are controlled by the Heart beating which is the basic motive force for Blood flow. As flow of Blood also depends on the propelling effect of Qi and Blood follows the ascending, descending, outgoing and entering movements of Qi to be distributed to the whole body, the Lung, which controls the Qi of the whole body and respiration and regulates the movement of Qi in the whole body, also plays a role in the distribution and regulation of Blood flow.

Assisting the Heart to govern the whole body is a summation of the Lung's main phyiological functions, which is mainly manifested as four aspects: firstly, the respiration is a rhythmical movement; secondly, the Lung's respiration controls and regulates flow of Qi in the whole body to ensure the normality of the ascending, descending, outgoing and entering movements of Qi; thirdly, the Lung can assist the Heart to propel and regulate flow of Blood through its ascending, descending, outgoing and entering movements; and fourthly, the Lung's dispersing and descending effects can control and regulate the distribution, flow and discharge of Body Fluid.

(2) Connections between the Lung and the emotions, secretions, body tissues and orifices:

① Related to sorrow in emotions: Both sorrow and anxiety are the unpleasant response of the body to the unfavorable stimuli of the external world, which often lead to constant consumption of Qi. As Qi is dominated by the Lung, sorrow or anxiety tends to impair the Lung. On the other hand, when the Lung is deficient, tolerance of the body to the unfavorable stimuli from the environment will decline, leading to liability to be in a state of sorrow or anxiety.

② Related to nasal discharge in secretions: The nasal discharge is the mucous fluid secreted from the nasal mucosa, which functions to moisten the nasal cavity. The nose is the orifice of the Lung, so the nasal discharge is related to the Lung. When the Lung Qi is sufficient, the nasal discharge can moisten the nasal cavity normally and does not flow out of the nose. Pathologically, Lung Cold often causes watery nasal discharge; Lung Heat often leads to yellow and sticky nasal discharge; and Lung Dryness often gives rise to inadequate nasal discharge and dry nose. Although the nose is the orifice of the Lung, it also communicates with the brain. So there is the saying that nasal discharge comes from the brain in *Huang Di Nei Jing* (The Yellow Emperor's Internal Classics).

③ Related to skin in body tissues and having its specific manifestations in hair: Skin and hair include the skin, sweat glands and vellus hairs here, which are the most superficial parts of the body. They depend on the defensive Qi and Body Fluid for their warmth and nourishment and serve as a barrier to prevent attack of exogenous pathogens. As the Lung can send defensive Qi as well as the Body Fluid and food essence to the skin and hairs, it is suggested in *Huang Di Nei Jing* (The Yellow Emperor's Internal Classics) that the Lung controls the skin and hairs. When the physiological functions of the Lung are normal, the skin will be compact, and the vellus hairs will be lustrous, thus they have a strong capacity to fight against invasion of exogenous pathogens. If the Lung Qi is deficient, its effect of sending defensive Qi and food essence to the skin and hairs will be weakened, as a result, the defensive Qi will fail to consolidate the surface of the body, manifested as polyhidrosis, liability to suffer from cold or withering of the skin and hairs. When exogenous pathogen attacks the skin and hairs, it often influences the Lung, leading to failure of the Lung Qi to disperse; while when the Lung Qi fails to disperse, it often causes closing of the striae of the muscles and stagnation of the defensive Qi.

In TCM, the sweat pore is also known as the gate of air, which means that the sweat pore not only has the effect of discharging sweat, but also has the effect of performing exchange of air together with the dispersing and descending effects of the Lung.

④ Opening into the nose: The nose is the passageway of the respiratory Qi and has a smelling function. As the Lung dominates respiration, the nose is the uppermost part of the respiratory tract and the Lung communicates with nature through the nose, it is said that the nose is the orifice of the Lung. The throat, like the nose, is also the gate of respiration, linking with both the nose and the Lung, so it is also said that the throat is the gate of the Lung. Therefore, the functional activities of both the nose and the throat depend on the dispersing of the Lung Qi. When the Lung functions properly, the respiration will be smooth, the smelling will be good and the voice will be high as a result of smooth flow of Qi through the throat. When exogenous pathogens attack the Lung, they often enter the Lung through the nose and throat. Or the other way round, Lung disorders often present manifestations of the nose and throat, such as nasal obstruction, nasal discharge, sneeze, itching of throat, hoarseness or aphonia.

3. The Spleen

The Spleen is located in the Middle Jiao below the diaphragm. It belongs to earth in Five Elements and its main functions are to transform and transport, to dominate up-sending of nutrients and to control Blood flow. Due to the connecting and pertaining of their meridians, the Spleen and the Stomach have an interior-exterior relationship with each other. The Spleen opens into the mouth, has its specific manifestations on the lips, is related to anxiety in emotions and the thick part of saliva and dominates the limbs and muscles.

(1) The main functions of the Spleen:

① Dominating transformation and transportation: This implies that the Spleen has the function of transforming food into essence and then distributing the essence to the whole body. This function of the Spleen can be divided into two aspects:

Dominating transformation and transportation of food: This means that the Spleen controls the digestion and absorption of foodstuff. Actually, the digestion and absorption of food are carried out in the Stomach and the Small Intestine, but transformation of food into the essence depends on the functional activity of the Spleen, and only through the transportation effect of the Spleen can the nutrients in the food essence be absorbed and sent to the whole body. When the Spleen has a strong effect of transforming and transporting food, the body's function in digestion and absorption of food will be good, thus essence, Qi, Blood and Body Fluid can be generated adequately and the Zang Fu organs, meridians, limbs and bones can be nourished sufficiently so that they can perform their normal physiological functions. Decline of the Spleen in transformation and transportation will cause abnormal digestion and absorption of the food, manifested as abdominal fullness, loose stools, poor appetite, or even lassitude, emaciation and inadequate production of Qi and Blood.

Transforming and transporting water: This refers to that the Spleen dominates absorption, distribution and discharge of water, which is an important link in water metabolism. This effect of the Spleen can absorb the surplus water and send it to the Lung and Kidney in time to be discharge in the form of sweat and urine under the steaming effects of the Lung and the Kidney. For this reason, if the transforming and transporting effect of the Spleen is strong, it can prevent abnormal retention of water in the body and thus avoid formation of such pathological products as Dampness and Phlegm. If the Spleen is unable to transform and transport water properly, water will accumulate in the body, leading to production of Dampness or Phlegm or even edema. This is just the mechanism of Deficiency of Spleen causing production of Dampness, the Spleen being the source for production of Phlegm and the edema caused by Spleen Deficiency.

The Spleen's functions of transforming and transporting food and water are inseparable from each other. They are both very important to the life activities of the human body. Man depends on Qi and Blood for his survival, whereas Qi and Blood depend on the food essence for their production, and the absorption of the food essence depends on the transforming or digesting effect of the Spleen and Stomach. So it is said that the Spleen and the Stomach are the sources for the production of Qi and Blood and serve as the basis of the acquired constitution of the human body. This is of great significance in the prevention and treatment of disease as well as in preserving health and preventing aging. For example, in treatment of a disease, food should be taken in accordance with the patient's condition and the medicines adopted should be good to the Spleen and the Stomach. Even in daily life, one should also take measures to protect his Spleen and Stomach. All these are the concrete manifestations of this theory in the prevention and treatment of disease and keeping health.

② Sending up nutrients: This means that the transforming and transporting effect of the Spleen is mainly reflected as its sending up nutrients. The Spleen Qi tends to go upwards, so it is said that the Spleen dominates ascending. Through the ascending movement of the Spleen Qi, food essence is sent to the Heart, the Lung, the head, the eyes, etc. , to produce Qi and Blood to nourish the whole body under the action of the Heart and the Lung. Therefore, there is the saying that the Spleen can function properly only when its Qi goes up. Ascending-descending movement is one kind of the movements of Qi of the Zang Fu organs. The effect of the Spleen in sending up nutrients is opposite to the effect of the Stomach in sending down the turbid substance. Sending up nutrients refers to absorption and distribution of food essence, while sending down the turbid means that the food residue is sent downwards gradually from the Stomach to the Small Intestine and then to the Large Intestine to be discharged in the form of faeces. In addition, coordinative and balanced ascending and descending movements of Qi of Zang Fu organs work as a main factor contributing to fixation of the visceral organs in proper positions. Therefore, ascending movement of the Spleen Qi, to some extent, has the effect of preventing prolapse of the internal organs. If the Spleen sends up nutrients properly, Qi and Blood can be generated adequately, the life activities can be well supported, and the visceral organs can be kept in their normal positions. If the Spleen fails to send up nutrients due to Spleen Qi Deficiency, inadequate production of Qi and Blood will give rise to such symptoms as listlessness, dizziness, lassitude, abdominal distention and diarrhea. If the Spleen Qi sinks instead of going upwards, it will cause such diseases as protracted diarrhea or even prolapse of the rectum, or prolapse of the visceral organs. Besides, failure of the Spleen Qi to ascend will also cause inability of the Stomach to send down the turbid, manifested as disturbance of the ascending-descending movement of Qi in the Middle Jiao.

③ Controlling normal flow of Blood: This means that the Spleen can keep Blood flowing in the meridians and prevent it from extravasation. This is mainly because Qi can control the normal flow of Blood and the Spleen serves as the source for production of Qi and Blood. When the Spleen's transforming and transporting effect is normal, Qi and Blood is sufficiently produced, thus Qi has a strong effect of controlling Blood flow. If the Spleen has a weak transformation and transportation, Qi and Blood will become deficient as a result of its inadequate production, thus the controlling effect of Qi is weakened and bleeding will occur. As the Spleen Qi dominates ascending, such diseases as hemafecia, hematuria and metrostaxis and metrorrhagia are usually regarded as the result of failure of the Spleen to keep normal flow of Blood.

(2) Connections of the Spleen with emotions, secretions, body tissues and orifices:

① Related to thinking in emotions: Thinking is one kind of emotional state which is related to both the Spleen and the function of the Heart in dominating spirit, so it is suggested that the thinking comes from the Heart and forms in the Spleen. As a normal mental activity, thinking usually exerts no unfavorable influence on the physiological activities of the human body. However, in the case of overthinking or failure to realize what one expects, it may influence the normal activities of the human body, especially the ascending, descending, outgoing and entering movements of Qi, leading to stagnation of Qi. Accumulation of Qi in the Middle Jiao again causes disturbance of the transforming and transporting function of the

51

Spleen, and the ensuing inadequate production of Qi and Blood, which is manifested initially as poor appetite, epigastric and abdominal fullness and distention and sighing, or even sallow complexion, dizziness, vertigo, palpitation, shortness of breath and forgetfulness, the symptoms of Deficiency of both the Heart and the Spleen, in severe cases.

② Related to saliva in secretions: Saliva is the clear part of the secretion of mouth, which functions to protect the mouth mucosa and moisten the mouth, thus it assists in swallowing and digestion of food. It is said in TCM that the saliva comes from the Spleen and flows up to the mouth from the Stomach. In normal circumstance, the saliva exists in the mouth instead of flowing out of the mouth. In the case of incoordination between the Stomach and the Spleen, sudden increase of the saliva will cause slobber, so the Spleen is related to saliva in secretions.

③ Related to muscles in body tissues and dominating the limbs: This means that whether the muscles are strong or whether the limbs act properly or not is closely related to the transforming and transporting effect of the Spleen. Since the Spleen and Stomach are the sources for the production of Qi and Blood, all the muscles of the body depend on food essence transformed and transported by the Spleen and Stomach for their nourishment so that they are well developed and robust. If the transforming and transporting effect of the Spleen and Stomach is disturbed, the muscles will be emaciated, weak or even atrophic. The limbs are the extremities of the human body and they also depend on the nourishment of the food essence transformed and transported by the Spleen and Stomach for their normal physiological activities. Therefore, when the Spleen has a strong transforming and transporting effect, the limbs will be well nourished and thus flexible and forceful. If the Spleen fails to transform and transport properly, the clear Yang will fail to be sent up and the nutrients will be to be distributed, which will further result in malnutrition of the limbs and the ensuing lassitude or even flaccidity of the limbs.

④ Opening into the mouth and having its specific manifestations on the lips: The mouth is the uppermost part of the digestive tract. That the Spleen opens into the mouth means that the appetite and taste in mouth are closely related to the transforming and transporting effect of the Spleen. Whether the taste in the mouth is normal or not is completely determined by the transforming and transporting effect of the Spleen and Stomach. If the Spleen can send up nutrients normally, the Stomach can send the turbid downward properly and the Spleen and Stomach have a strong transforming and transporting effect, the taste in the mouth and the appetite will be normal. If the Spleen loses its transforming and transporting effect, poor appetite and flat taste in the mouth will occur. In the case of Damp Heat in the Spleen, there will be sweat taste or sticky taste in the mouth. If Fire or Heat accumulates in the Spleen, it may go upwards along with the Spleen channel to cause mouth ulcer or erosion.

The colour and the luster of the lips are related to the vicissitude of Qi and Blood of the whole body. As the Spleen is where Qi and Blood are generated, whether the lips are ruddy or lustrous can reflect the functional state of the Spleen and Stomach in transforming and transporting the food essence. Thus, in *Wu Zang Sheng Cheng* (Formation of the Five Zang Organs) in *Su Wen* (The Plain Questions), it is stated that "The Spleen connects with muscles and can be reflected on the lips."

4. The Liver

The Liver is located in the right hypochondrium below the diaphragm in the abdominal cavity. It belongs to wood in the Five Elements and tends to be active and go upwards. In Chapter of *Ling Lan Mi Dian Lun* (Extremely Important Treatise) in *Su Wen* (The Plain Questions), it is described as a General Organ. The main functions of the Liver are to dominate dispersing and discharging and store Blood. The Liver opens into the eyes, has its specific manifestations in the nails, dominates tendons, is related to anger in emotions and tear in secretions. As the Liver links with the Gallbladder and their channels belong to or connect with these two organs respectively, these two organs have an interior-exterior relationship.

(1) The main functions of the Liver:

① Dominating dispersing and discharging: This means that the Liver has the effect of dispersing and discharging Qi, Blood and Body Fluid so that they can flow and be discharged smoothly. This is a reflection of such physiological features of the Liver as being a rigid organ, going upwards and actively. The dispersing and discharging effect of the Liver is mainly manifested as three aspects:

Soothing flow of Qi and promoting circulation of Blood and Body Fluid: The functional activities of the Zang Fu organs of the human body depend on the ascending, descending, outgoing and entering movements of Qi. Since the Liver dominates ascending and discharging movements in physiology, it plays an important role in promoting Qi to flow smoothly and upward. The dispersing and discharging effect of the Liver has a regulatory effect on the balance and coordination of the ascending, descending, outgoing and entering of Qi. If the Liver functions properly in its dispersing and discharging effect, Qi and Blood will be kept in harmony, the meridians will be unobstructed and the functional activities of the Zang Fu organs will be normal and coordinated. If this effect of the Liver is disturbed, it often causes two kinds of pathological changes: decline of the Liver's dispersing and discharging effect, which will give rise to inadequate ascending of Qi and obstruction of flow of Qi, sluggish flow of Qi or stagnation of Qi, manifested as distending pain in such local areas as the breasts, hypochondrium and the bilateral sides of the lower abdomen; and excessive ascending of the Liver, which causes excessive ascending and inadequate descending movement of Qi, resulting in rising of the Liver Qi that is marked by distending pain in the head, red face and eyes and irritability. In the case of excessive rising of Qi, Blood may follow Qi to go upwards, leading to hematemesis or hemoptysis, or even sudden coma due to disorder of Qi.

Circulation of Blood and distribution of Body Fluid both depend on the ascending, descending, outgoing and entering movements of Qi. As the Liver dominates dispersion and discharge, it can regulate flow of Qi and thus promote the flow of Blood and Body Fluid.

Stagnation of Qi will cause Blood Stasis as a result of stagnation of Blood or Phlegm due to retention of Body Fluid, or even abdominal masses and other diseases caused by combination of the stagnated Qi with Blood Stasis or with Phlegm. In addition, bleeding may occur in the case of excessive rising of Qi as a result of Blood rushing out of the vessels.

Promoting the transforming and transporting effect of the Spleen and the Stomach: The function of the Spleen and Stomach in transformation and transportation is closely related to the dispersing and discharging effect of the Liver. On the one hand, the Liver's dispersing and discharging effect can regulate movements of Qi, which is beneficial to the balance and coordination between the sending-up-nutrient effect of the Spleen and the sending-down-turbid effect of the Stomach and ensure the normal performance of the transforming and transporting effect of the Spleen and Stomach. If the Liver's dispersing and discharging effect is disturbed, it may cause such pathological changes as encroachment of the excessive wood on the earth, leading to disturbance of the Spleen's function of sending up nutrients and the ensuing occurrence of such Syndromes as attack of the Liver Qi on the Spleen or inccordination between the Liver and the Spleen, which is marked by vomiting or hiccup in the upper part of the body, epigastric and abdominal fullness in the middle and constipation in the lower. On the other hand, the Liver's dispersing and discharging influence the secretion and excretion of the bile directly, and thus influence the transforming and transporting effect of the Spleen and the Stomach. The Gallbladder is linked up with the Liver, and in accordance with TCM theory, the bile comes from accumulation of the residue part of the Liver Qi. Thus the secretion and excretion of bile are in fact a part of the function of the Liver's dispersing and discharging effect. When the Liver has a normal dispersing and discharging effect, the bile will be secreted and excreted normally so that it can assist the Spleen and Stomach in their transformating and transporting foodstuff. If the Liver Qi stagnates and thus the secretion and excretion of bile are disturbed, it will cause poor appetite, distention or pain in the hypochondriac region, bitter taste in the mouth, disinclination to eat greasy or fatty food, or even jaundice.

Regulating the emotions: The emotional states are a part of the spirit controlled by the Heart, but they are also closely related to the Liver, because the normal emotional states depend on free flow of Qi and Blood which is dredged by the Liver's dispersing and discharging effect. The most important influence of emotional disturbance, on the other hand, lies in that it may disturb the normal flow of Qi and Blood. Therefore, when the Liver performs its dispersing and discharging effect properly, Qi will flow smoothly, Qi and Blood will be coordinated and thus one has ease of mind and is cheerful. If the Liver's dispersing and discharging effect declines, it will cause stagnation of the Liver Qi which is often marked by mental depression and liability to become sorrow or anxious. If the Liver's dispersing and discharging effect is excessive, the Liver Qi or the Liver Fire may rise, leading to irritability. Conversely, repeated or persistent emotional disturbance will give rise to disturbance of the Liver's dispersing and discharging effect, thus such pathological changes as stagnation of the Liver Qi or excessive rising of the Liver Qi will occur.

In addition, ovulation and menstruation in females and ejaculation in males are also closely related to the dispersing and discharging effect of the Liver. Clinically, regulating the Liver serves as the most important method in treatment of irregular menstruation, so there is the saying that females take the Liver as the basis of their congenital constitution.

② Storing Blood: This indicates that the Liver has a function of storing Blood and regulating the Blood volume, which is mainly manifested as four aspects:

The Liver belongs to Yin in structure and Yang in function, so it must store certain amount of Blood to restrict the ascending of the Liver Yang to prevent it from rising excessively, thereby maintaining the normal dispersing and discharging of the Liver. If the Liver fails to store Blood, inadequate storage of Blood in the Liver will cause Deficiency of the Liver Blood, or as a result of failure of the

Liver Yang to be restricted, causing such pathological changes as hyperactivity of the Liver Yang, flaring up of the Liver Fire and stirring of the Liver Wind.

The storage of Blood in the Liver has the effect of preventing bleeding. If the Liver cannot store Blood, pathological changes marked by bleeding such as hematemesis, epistaxis or metrostaxis and metrorrhagia may be noted.

That the Liver stores Blood plays an important role in the adjustment of the peripheral Blood volume, as it can regulate assignment of Blood in different parts of the body. Under normal conditions, the Blood volumes in different parts of the body are relatively stable, but they vary with changes of the body's activities, emotions and climatic conditions. In the case of violent physical activities or emotional upset, the Liver sends the Blood it stores to the peripheral tissues of the body to meet the needs of the body. Conversely, when one is on rest or in a stable emotional state, the peripheral tissues need less Blood as a result of reduce of the activities of the body, thus part of the Blood flows to the Liver to be stored. It should be pointed that the function of Liver in regulating Blood volume takes the functions of Liver storing Blood as its basis. Only when enough Blood is stored in the Liver can the Liver perform its function of regulating the Blood volume. In fact, the function of the Liver distributing the Blood it stores to the peripheral tissues is an aspect of the Liver's dispersing and discharging effect in Blood circulation. So, the Blood stored in the Liver can be distributed to the peripheral tissues normally only when the Liver conducts its dispersing and discharging effect regularly and thus the Blood flows smoothly. For these reasons, the function of the Liver in regulating Blood volume depends on the coordinative balance of the dispersing and discharging effect of the Liver and the function of storing Blood. If the Liver Qi ascends excessively or it fails to store Blood, various kinds of bleeding will ensue. When the Liver fails to disperse and discharge, the Liver Qi will stagnate and so Blood Stasis will follow.

The effect of the Liver in storing Blood and regulating Blood volume can regulate and control the occurrence of menstruation to keep the menses normal in colour, quality and volume. So, Deficiency of the Liver Blood or failure of the Liver to store Blood may cause hypomenorrhea or even amenorrhea, menorrhagia, metrorrhagia or metrostaxis.

Since the Liver stores Blood and regulates Blood volume, physiological functions of different parts of the human body are all related to the Liver. In the case of inability of the Liver to store Blood due to Liver disorder, it will not only cause Blood Deficiency or bleeding, but also cause diseases marked by malnutrition of Blood in the different parts of the body. For example, failure of Blood to nourish the eyes will cause blurred vision, dry eyes, or night blindness, failure of the Liver Blood to nourish the tendons will cause convulsion, numbness of limbs and difficulty of the limbs in flexion and extension, etc.

In addition, there is the saying of the Liver storing soul in viscera-state theory. The soul is a mental activity secondary to spirit. As stated in *Ben Shen* (The Primordial Spirit) of *Ling Shu* (The Miraculous Pivat): "That comes and goes with spirit is called soul." Just like the spirit, the soul also takes Blood as its material basis. As the Heart dominates Blood, it houses spirit. As the Liver stores Blood, it stores soul. When the Liver has a strong effect of storing Blood, the soul has a place to be stored. If the Liver Blood is deficient and the Heart Blood is depleted, soul will be unable to be stored, so there is dream-disturbed sleep, insomnia, sleeping walking, somniloquy or hallucination.

(2) Connections of the Liver with the emotions, secretions, body tissues and orifices:

① Related to anger in emotions: Anger is an emotional state occurring in the case of excitement. As disturbance of the Liver's dispersing and discharging effect often leads to irritability and over-anger is most likely to impair the Liver, it is considered that the anger is related to the Liver. In most cases, anger exerts unfavorable influence on the physiological activities. The ancient Chinese believed that anger occurring in the case of something unpleasant is a normal response of the body in mental activities. However, sudden and violent rage or repeated attack of anger may cause the excessive ascending of the Liver Yang and thus impair the Liver. The main influence of anger on the human body is that it can cause adverse upward flow of Qi, even ascending of Blood following the Qi to cause sudden hematemesis and sudden syncope, and diarrhea due to failure of the Spleen to send up nutrients. Or the other way round, Deficiency of the Liver Yin or the Liver Blood, excessive rising of the Liver Qi or flaring up of the Liver Fire, often causes irritability.

② Related to tear in secretions: Tear has the function of moistening, nourishing and protecting the eyes. As it is secreted from the eyes and the eyes are the orifices of the Liver, it is said that the Liver is related to tear in secretions. Under normal conditions, the tear secreted can moisten the eyeball and keep it clean. When foreign body enters the eye, tear will be secreted massively so as to clean the eyeballs and get rid of the foreign body. In pathological conditions, abnormal secretion of tear is often encountered in the case of Deficiency of Yin Blood of the Liver which often leads to reduce of the secretion of tear, manifested as dry eyes, or in the case of Dampness Heat in the Liver meridian or upward attack of the Wind Fire, which often causes the increased secretion of tear, manifested as lacrimation or tearing on aversion to wind. In addition, when one is extremely sorrow, the tear may also be secreted in a large amount.

③ Related to tendon in body tissues and having its specific manifestations on nails: Tendons, attached to bones and meeting around joints, is a kind of tissues connecting the joints and muscles. As a result of the contraction and extension of the tendons, the joints exhibit various movements, and as the movements of the tendons depend on the nourishment of the Liver Blood, it is said that the Liver is related to tendons in body tissues. If the Liver has a strong effect of storing Blood and controlling dispersing and discharging, the tendons will be strenous, vigorous and tolerant to tiredness. If the tendons lose nourishment due to Deficiency of the Liver Blood or stagnation of the Liver Qi, their moving ability will decline, leading to tremor of the hands and feet, numbness of the limbs, difficulty of the limbs in extension and reflexion or even convulsion. Therefore, it is stated in *Huang Di Nei Jing* (The Yellow Emperor's Internal Classics) that the Liver is the basis of bearing tiredness and the Liver dominates tendons.

Nails refer to those of both the hands and the feet, which are considered to be remainder of the tendons in TCM. Luster of the nails depends on the nourishment of the Liver Blood, hence the saying that the Liver has its specific manifestation the nails. When the Liver Blood is sufficient, the nails will be sturdy, lustrous and ruddy, while if the Liver Blood is deficient, the nails will be thin, withered and lustreless, or even deformed and cracked.

④ Opening into the eyes: Eyes, also known as "brightness of essence", are the visual organs. They are related to the Liver because the Liver channel connects upwards with the eye systems and the vision depends on nourishment of the Liver Blood and propelling of the dispersing and discharging effect of the Liver. However, all the essence Qi of the Five Zang organs and the Six Fu organs go up to the eyes, so the eyes are also related to all these organs. As the Liver has a close relationship with the eyes, functional states of the Liver can be reflected on the eyes. For example, when the Liver Blood is deficient, the eyes will be dry with blurred vision or night blindness. When Wind Heat attacks the Liver channel, there are usually redness, itching and pain of the eyes. In the case of flaring up of the Liver Fire, the eyes may become blood-shot with nebula. If the Liver Yang rises excessively, there will be dizziness and vertigo. And if the Liver Wind stirs inside, it may cause strabismus or up-staring of the eyes.

5. The Kidney

The Kidneys are located in the lumbar region beside the spinal column, each on either side. As the Kidneys are located in the lumbar region, it is said in *Mai Yao Jing Wei Lun* (Treatise on Highlights of Taking Pulse) in *Su Wen* (The Plain Questions) that the lumbar region houses the Kidneys. The Kidney is where the congenital essence is stored, so it is the basis of Yin and Yang of the Zang

Fu organs and the source of life, and thus the Kidney is also called the basis of the congenital constitution of the human body. In the Five Elements, the Kidney belongs to water and its main physiological functions are to store essence, dominate growth, development and reproduction, and control water metabolism. Besides, the Kidney governs bones, in charge of generation of marrow, has its specific manifestations on hair, opens into the external genital and the anus as well as the ears. In emotional states, it is related to terror and fright, and in secretions, it is related to spittle. As the Kidney channel and the Bladder channel pertain to and connect with the Kidney and the Bladder respectively and the Kidney is directly related to the Bladder in water metabolism, the Kidney and the Bladder have an interior-exterior relationship.

(1) The main functions of the Kidney:

① Dominating storage: This means that the Kidney has the physiological effect of receiving, storing and keeping the essence. This effect can keep the essence storing in the Kidney to maintain the fulfill of the Kidney essence and prevent useless loss of the essence so that the essence Qi can perform its physiological effect in the body regularly. Under normal circumstances, as a result of the storing effect of the Kidney, the Kidney essence is constantly supplemented to be kept in a stable amount so that it can maintain the health of the body. If the Kidney's storing effect declines, it may cause useless discharge of the essence or inadequate supplement of the Kidney essence, leading to Deficiency of the Kidney essence. Therefore, the storing effect of the Kidney is an important content of the physiological function of the Kidney in storing essence.

② Dominating growth, development and reproduction: Essence is a basic substance constituting the human body and maintaining its normal life activities. The essence has two meanings: in a broad sense, it refers to the refined parts of any substances which have a strong nourishing effect, such as Qi, Blood, Body Fluid and the food essence absorbed from food; in a narrow sense, it indicates the reproductive essence, including the productive essence inherited from parents. The essence stored in the Kidney refers to neither the

61

mere productive essence inherited from parents nor the essence of the broad sense. It has its specific meanings, so it is generally referred to as the essence Qi of the Kidney, which can be classified as two components in accordance with their different sources, the congenital essence and the acquired essence after birth. The former indicates the productive essence inherited from parents which exists at the very beginning of life and serves as the primordial substance for the formation of embryo; while the latter refers to the food essence transformed by the Spleen after one's birth and the residue part of the essence produced in the Zang Fu organs. Although they come from different sources, these two kinds of essence coexist in the Kidney and depend on and supplement each other. The congenital essence depends on the constant nourishment of the acquired essence after birth for the full performance of its physiological effect, while the acquired essence after birth depends on assistance of the vitality from the congenital essence for its generation and absorption. So, they supplement each other in the Kidney to compose of the Kidney essence.

The main physiological functions of the Kidney essence are to promote the growth and development of the human body and the gradual formation of the reproductive ability. In one's whole life, his kidney essence enjoys a process of changing from weak to strong and then from strong to weak or to dismiss. The vicissitude of the Kidney essence controls the generation, growth, aging and death of the human life. In *Shang Gu Tian Zhen Lun* (On Innate Essence) in *Su Wen* (The Plain Questions), it is clearly pointed out that in the adolescence after one's birth, the Kidney essence gradually becomes full and gives rise to such changes of growing of hair and the exchange of teeth. With the continuous filling of the Kidney essence, *Tiangui*, a refined substance with the function of promoting the development of sexual glands, is produced, which causes the maturity of the sexual glands and the coming of the adolescent period. As a result, female begins to have ovulation and menstruation, and male begins to have emissions, so both the female and male have the reproductive capacity. When one is middle aged, with the gradual decline of the Kidney essence, *Tiangui* turns to be reduced or exhausted, as a result, the sexual ability as well as the reproductive ability decline gradually, and the body physique also shows signs of aging which means that the senile period is coming.

The Kidney essence is the basis of the life activities. It plays a leading role in the physiological functions of the human body. Through ages, doctors have made plenty of studies on the Kidney essence and their effects on the life activities. In order to expound the physiological effect of the Kidney essence completely in both theory and clinical practice, the effect of the Kidney essence is generalized as two aspects: that functioning to nourishing and moistening the Zang Fu organs and tissues is referred to as the Kidney Yin, while that functioning to propel and warm the Zang Fu organs and tissues, as the Kidney Yang. Both the Kidney Yin and the Kidney Yang take the essence Qi stored in the Kidney as their material basis. The Kidney Yin and the Kidney Yang, also known as the genuine Yin or genuine Yang, or the true Yin and the true Yang, serve as basis of the Yin and Yang of Zang Fu organs. They restrict each other, depend on each other and assist each other, maintaining the relative balance of Yin and Yang of the Zang Fu organs. If, for some reasons, the relative balance between the Kidney Yin and the Kidney Yang is disturbed, imbalance of Yin Yang of the Kidney will occur, manifested as either Kidney Yin Deficiency or Kidney Yang Deficiency. Kidney Yin Deficiency is often manifested as tidal fever, night sweat, dizziness, tinnitus, soreness and weakness of the loins and knees, nocturnal emission in male or sexual intercourse in dream in females, red and less moistened tongue; while Kidney Yang Deficiency, as listlessness, cold pain in the loins and knees, cold limbs and aversion to cold, frequent urination, pale tongue and impotence or premature ejaculation in male and sterility due to uterus Cold in female.

Disturbance of Yin and Yang of Zang Fu organs often occurs following disturbance of Yin and Yang of the Kidney, because the Kidney Yin and the Kidney Yang are the basis of the Yin and Yang of Zang Fu organs. For example, when the Liver loses the nourishment of the Kidney Yin, which is known as failure of water to nourish the wood, it may lead to hyperactivity of the Liver Yang or even stirring up of the Liver Wind; failure of the Kidney Yin to nourish the Heart Yin may cause flaring up of the Heart Fire or Deficiency of both the Kidney Yin and the Heart Yin; inability of the Kidney Yin to nourish the Lung Yin often gives rise to Deficiency of both the Lung Yin and the Kidney Yin; failure of the Kidney Yang to warm the Heart Yang often causes Deficiency of both the Kidney Yang and the Heart Yang; and inability of the Kidney Yang to warm the Spleen Yang often causes Deficiency of both the Kidney Yang and the Spleen Yang. Conversely, Deficiency of Yin or Yang of other Zang Fu organs will affect the Kidney Yin or the Kidney Yang if lasting a long time, consuming the essence Qi of the Kidney and leading to disturbance of the Kidney Yin and the Kidney Yang, which is generally called protracted diseases affecting the Kidney.

③ Dominating water metabolism: This means that the Kidney plays an important role in maintaining the balance of water metabolism through controlling distribution and discharge of water, so the Kidney is also called a water organ. This effect of the Kidney is mainly carried out by the steaming effect of the Kidney essence. In normal conditions, the Body Fluid fulfills its metabolism by the receiving effect of the Stomach, the transforming and transporting effect of the Spleen, the dispersing and descending effect of the Lung, and the steaming effect of the Kidney with the Triple Jiao as its passageway. The metabolized water is discharged out of the body in the form of sweat, urine, etc. Thus, water metabolism is a complicated physiological process in which many Zang Fu organs play different roles. Of these effects of Zang Fu organs, the steaming effect of the Kidney exists in the whole course of water metabolism. Such effects as the Lung's dispersing and the ascending and the distributing effect of the Spleen, all depend on propelling of the steaming and vapourizing effect of the Kidney. The formation and discharge of urine which plays an extremely important part in maintaining the balance of water metabolism of the body, in particular, is more closely related to the steaming and vapourizing effect of the

Kidney. Therefore, it is said in TCM that the Kidney dominates water metabolism. When the essence Qi of the Kidney declines, its steaming effect will become weak, as a result, the steaming effects of the Spleen, the Lung and the Triple Jiao will be disturbed, and the closing-opening effect of the Kidney and the Bladder will be destroyed, leading to oliguria, retention of urine, edema, or massive watery urine, increase of the urine volume, etc.

④ Dominating reception of Qi: This indicates that the Kidney has an effect of receiving the fresh air inhaled by the Lung to prevent breathing from becoming shollow. Although it is the Lung that dominates respiration, breathing also depends on the reception effect of the Kidney to carry out the normal exchange of air both inside and outside the body. So, there is the saying that the Lung is the master of Qi while the Kidney is the root of Qi. The effect of the Kidney in receiving Qi is in fact a manifestation of the storing effect of the Kidney in respiration. In the light of TCM theory, the fresh air inhaled by the Lung must go down to the Kidney and thus the depth of breathing mainly depends on the receiving effect of the Kidney. When the Kidney receives Qi properly, respiration will be even and coordinative. If the Kidney Qi is deficient, it will fail to receive air, leading to shallow breathing, long exhalation and short inhalation or dyspnea on even slight exertion, which is known as failure of the Kidney to receive air.

(2) Connections of the Kidney with the emotions, secretions, body tissues and orifices:

① Related to terror in emotions: Terror is a kind of emotional state marked by timidiness. It is similar to fright, but fright is often caused by external stimuli, while terror is often the result of internal disorders. Both of them will cause unfavorable stimuli to the human body and are considered to be related to the Kidney. Apart from the Kidney, terror is also related to the Heart which controls mental activity. When the spirit housed by the Heart is impaired, one will become timid and tend to be terror. Since both terror and fright are the responses based on the functional activities of the Kidney, sudden terror or fright often injures the Kidney, leading to collapse of Qi or disturbance of flow of Qi. This means that in the state of terror, the Upper Jiao is obstructed and Qi is forced to flow to the Lower Jiao, causing abdominal fullness or even incontinence of urination and defecation. When sudden fright impairs the body, Qi cannot flow to the Heart to support the Heart spirit, as a result, one will be disattracted and alarmed.

② Related to spittle in secretions: Spittle refers to the thick part of the saliva. TCM believes that the spittle comes from the Kidney essence. In normal conditions, it should be swallowed instead of being spitted to nourish the Kidney essence. If one spits too much or frequently, his Kidney essence is likely to be impaired. So, experts in health preservation in ancient China advocated that the Kidney essence may be nourished by supporting the upper palate with one's tongue to promote secretion of the spittle and then swallowing the spittle slowly when it fills the mouth. Although spittle is the secretion related to the Kidney, it also has something to do with the Spleen and the Stomach, so frequent spittle may be seen in both patients with Kidney Deficiency and those with Deficiency of the Stomach Yang just after a severe disease.

③ Related to bone in body tissues, dominating bone and generating marrow and having its specific manifestations in the hair: The physiological effect of the Kidney in dominating bone and generating marrow is in fact a component part of the function of the Kidney essence in promoting the growth and development of the human body. The growth and development of bone depend on enough marrow filling with the bone and the nutrients provided by the marrow, while the bone marrow can be nourished only when the Kidney essence is replete. Therefore, it is considered that such disorders as delayed closure of the frontanel, weakness of bones and osteroporosis or liability of the bone to be fractured in the aged are all related to insufficiency of the bone marrow due to Deficiency of the essence Qi of the Kidney.

Marrow can be divided into three kinds, the bone marrow, the spinal marrow and the brain marrow, all of which are produced by the essence Qi of the Kidney. For this reason, vicissitude of the essence Qi of the Kidney not only influences the growth and development of bones, but also influences the filling and development of the spinal marrow and the brain marrow. The spinal marrow communicates with the brain upwards to meet there to form the brain marrow, hence the saying that the brain is the sea of marrow. When the essence Qi of the Kidney is sufficient, the "sea of marrow" will be well nourished, thus the brain is well developed and one is full of energy, strenuous and flexible in movements, has a good vision and hearing and a quick thinking. If the Kidney essence is deficient, listlessness, tinnitus, dizziness, slow thinking and soreness and weakness of the loins and knees, the signs of emptiness of the sea of marrow due to poor nourishment, will occur.

The teeth are the remainder of the bone, or both the bone and teeth are from the same source. So, growth and hardness of teeth also depend on nourishment of the Kidney essence. In the case of sufficiency of the Kidney essence, the teeth will be sturdy and will not be so easily shaked or fall. However, when the Kidney essence is deficient, the teeth will be easily shaked or fall earlier. As both the Large Intestine Channel of Hand-Yangming and the Stomach Channel of Foot-Yangming enter the teeth and go around the mouth, some disorders of the teeth are also related to the disturbance of the physiological functions of the Large Intestine and the Stomach.

The Kidney stores essence which can transform into Blood to nourish the hair. Sufficient essence will produce enough Blood to nourish the hair and thus the hair will be black and bright, so it is said that the Kidney has its specific manifestations on the hair. The vitality of hair comes from the Kidney, while its nourishment depends on the Blood, so there is the saying that the hair is the remainder of Blood. In the young and the middle aged, the hair is usually lustrous and bright as the Kidney essence and Blood are exuberant, while in the aged, it often turns to be grey and falls as a result of decline of the essence and Blood. Clinically, withering of hair or grey-turning or fall of hair are mostly caused by Deficiency of the Kidney essence and Deficiency of Blood.

④ Opening into the ears and the external genital and anus: The ear is an auditary organ and whether the hearing is good or not is closely related to the vicissitude of the Kidney essence, so it is considered that the ear is the orifice of the Kidney. Sufficiency of the Kidney essence will ensure the well nourishment of the brain and thus the hearing is good. If the Kidney essence is deficient, decline of hearing, tinnitus or even deafness are likely to occur due to loss of nourishment of the brain. In the aged people, the Kidney essence naturally becomes less, so their hearing is usually poor. Clinically, changes of hearing may be a sign of vicissitude of the Kidney essence.

The external genital is the organ controlling urination and reproductive activity, while the anus is where the faeces are discharged. Although discharge of urine is the function of the Bladder, it depends on the steaming effect of the Kidney to be performed, and the reproductive activity of the human body is also controlled by the Kidney. Besides, although the discharge of the faeces is mainly conducted by the transporting effect of the Large Intestine, it is also related to the steaming effect of the Kidney. When the Kidney Yin is deficient, Body Fluid in the Large Intestine will be exhausted, as a result, constipation will occur; in the case of Kidney Yang Deficiency, the Kidney will not be able to steam and thus constipation or diarrhea due to Yang Deficiency will occur; and if the Kidney fails to perform its storing effect, there may be protracted diarrhea or prolapse of the rectum, so the Kidney opens into the external genital and the anus.

The Six Fu Organs

The Six Fu organs refer to the Gallbladder, the Stomach, the Large Intestine, the Small Intestine, the Triple Jiao and the Bladder. Fu in Chinese means a house. The common physiological features of the Six Fu organs are to digest or ripen foodstuff and transport and discharge food residues. Food from their entering the mouth till their residues being discharged out of the body must pass through seven gates, which are known as the seven rushing gates of the digestive tract in *Nan Jing* (The Difficult Classics). That is, the door leaf, which is formed by the upper and lower lips, the meeting gate formed by the upper and lower teeth, the breathing gate formed by the epiglottis, the cardia or the upper opening of the Stomach, the pylorus or the lower opening of the Stomach, the blocking gate connecting the Small Intestine and the Large Intestine and the gate of soul or anus. Diseases of any of the seven gates will influence the receiving, digesting, absorbing and discharging of the foodstuff.

As the Six Fu organs function to transform and transport foodstuff, they are said to be filled with foodstuff instead of nutrients, and they can function properly when they work downward and the digestive tract is kept unblocked. If they work downwards without obstruction of the digestive tract, digestion will be normal, while if the digestive tract is blocked, diseases will ensue as a result.

1. The Gallbladder

The Gallbladder is both one of the Six Fu organs and an extraordinary organ. As its main function is to store and discharge bile to aid digestion of foodstuff, it is regarded as one of the Six Fu organs; but as the Gallbladder does not transform and transport the foodstuff itself, different from the Stomach and intestines, it is also considered to be an extraordinary organ. In structure, it links with the Liver and is attached to the short lobe of the Liver, and because of the pertaining-connecting relationships between their channels, the Gallbladder and the Liver have an interior-exterior relationship. In addition, it is also considered in the viscera-state theory that the Gallbladder dominates determination and judgment.

(1) Storing and discharging bile: Bile is a yellow-green and bitter liquid formed in the Liver and stored in the Gallbladder. When it is discharged into the Small Intestine, it can assist the digestion of foodstuff, thus it is an important condition for the normal performance of the digestive function of the Spleen and the Stomach. As

the bile comes from the Liver and is a clear fluid, the Gallbladder is also known as a clear organ in *Huang Di Nei Jing* (The Yellow Emperor's Internal Classics).

Apart from the bile being formed by the essence Qi of the Liver, its discharge is also controlled and regulated by the dispersing and discharging effect of the Liver. When the Liver's dispersing and discharging effect is normal, the bile will be discharged freely and so the transforming and transporting effect of the Spleen and the Stomach is strong. If the Liver fails to disperse or discharge, causing stagnation of the Liver Qi, failure of the bile to be discharged freely will cause disturbance of the transforming and transporting effect of the Spleen and the Stomach, giving rise to hypochondriac fullness and pain, poor appetite, abdominal fullness, loose stool, etc. If the Liver Qi ascends too much or the Liver Fire flares up, bile may go upward adversely, leading to hypochondriac fullness and pain, bitter taste in the mouth or even vomiting of yellow-green fluid. If the bile flows outwards, it may cause jaundice. Conversely, disturbance of discharge of bile due to other causes may influence the dispersing and discharging effect of the Liver, leading to diseases of the Liver.

(2) Dominating determination and judgment: As suggested in *Huang Di Nei Jing* (The Yellow Emperor's Internal Classics), this indicates that the Gallbladder is capable of doing judgment and then determining the measures to be adopted. It is also one kind of mental activities. In the clinic today, this function is not so often mentioned. It is generally believed that when he has sufficiency of the Gallbladder Qi, one will be brave and decisive; while he will be indecisive, timid, and alarmed if the Gallbladder Qi is deficient.

2. The Stomach

The Stomach can be divided into three parts: the upper, the middle and the lower. The upper part of the Stomach is also known as the Upper Wan, including the cardia, the middle part is also known as the Middle Wan, referring to the gastrict body mainly, and the lower part is also known as the Lower Wan, which includes the pylorus. The main functions of the Stomach are to receive and ripen foodstuff, and it tends to function downwards. Occasionally, the

70

functions of the Large Intestine and the Small Intestine are also included in the functions of the Stomach in *Huang Di Nei Jing* (The Yellow Emperor's Internal Classics).

(1) Dominating receiving and ripening of foodstuff: "Receiving" here means that the Stomach can receive food from the esophagus and then allow the food to stay for some time in the Stomach; while "ripening" means that the food in the Stomach is changed into the chyme through the primary digestion of the Stomach. As food is housed in the Stomach, the Stomach is also known as the sea of foodstuff or a greater barn. The physiological functions of the body as well as the generation of Qi, Blood and Body Fluid all depend on the foodstuff received and stored by the Stomach, so the Stomach is also known as the sea of water, food, Qi and Blood.

The food housed in the Stomach is sent to the Small Intestine after being primarily digested. The refined part is then absorbed and distributed by the Spleen's transforming and transporting function. In this process, the receiving and ripening function of the Stomach and the transforming and transporting effect of the Spleen play a leading role in the transformation of food and water into essence and the generation of Qi, Blood and Body Fluid, so the Spleen and Stomach are also called the basis of acquired constitution. In some cases, the receiving, ripening, transforming and transporting effects of the Spleen and Stomach are generally referred to as the Stomach Qi, vicissitude of which determines the life activities or the survival of the human body, so there is the saying that the life takes the Stomach Qi as its basis; and that one will be alive if he had Stomach Qi, and one will die if his Stomach Qi is absent. In the diagnosis and treatment of disease, taking care of the Stomach Qi must be regarded as an important principle for health preservation and treatment of diseases.

(2) Functioning downwards and with downward and unblocked movement of the Stomach Qi as its functional basis: The Stomach is the sea of food and water. Entering the Stomach and being primarily digested by the Stomach, the water and food must be sent down to the Small Intestine to be digested further, so the Stomach functions

71

downwards with downward and unblocked movement of the Stomach Qi as its functional basis. In the viscera-state theory, the physiological functions of the digestive tract of the human body can be generalized as the ascending movement of the Spleen Qi and the descending movement of the Stomach Qi. In addition, the descending function of the Stomach also includes the down-sending of the food residues from the Small Intestine to the Large Intestine and the transporting effect of the Large Intestine.

The Stomach mainly sends down the turbid substance, which is the prerequisite for the receiving effect of the Stomach. Normal descending of the Stomach Qi will ensure the downward going of food and thus the receiving effect of the Stomach can be normally performed. If the Stomach Qi fails to descend, there will be poor appetite or fetid odour in the mouth, fullness, distention or even pain in the epigastric region and abdomen and constipation due to accumulation of the turbid substance in the upper part. If failure of the Stomach in descending turbid causes upward adverse flow of the Stomach Qi, it may lead to eructation with sour odour, nausea, vomiting or hiccup.

3. The Small Intestine

The Small Intestine is a very long tube organ located in the abdominal cavity with its upper part connecting with the Stomach through the pylorus and its lower part connecting with the Large Intestine through the blocking gate. Its main functions are to receive and transform foodstuff and separate the nutrients from the waste.

(1) Receiving, housing and digesting foodstuff: The receiving and housing effect of the Small Intestine is mainly manifested as two aspects: firstly, the Small Intestine is a "container", receiving the foodstuff primarily digested from the Stomach; secondly, the foodstuff that has been digested primarily in the Stomach has to stay in the Small Intestine for a long time so that it is further digested and absorbed. The transforming effect of the Small Intestine means that the Small Intestine can further digest the foodstuff to turn it into food essence.

(2) Separating the nutrients from the waste: This is mainly mani-

fested as three aspects: firstly, the foodstuff digested in the Small Intestine is separated into two parts, the nutrients and the waste; secondly, the Small Intestine absorbs the nutrients and sends down the food residues to the Large Intestine; and thirdly, the Small Intestine also absorbs plenty of water while absorbing the nutrients, hence the saying that the Small Intestine controls fluid. Besides, this function is also related to the urine volume. When the Small Intestine can perform its effect, both urination and defecation will be normal. If the Small Intestine fails to separate the nutrients from the waste, there will be loose stool with scanty urine. So, in the clinic, such therapeutic method as inducing diuresis to treat diarrhea is often adopted.

The functional activities of the Small Intestine are very important to the transformation of foodstuff into the food essence and can be regarded as a concrete manifestation of the functions of the Spleen and Stomach in sending up nutrients and sending down the waste. Disturbance of the functional activities of the Small Intestine often causes abdominal fullness and pain, vomiting and constipation due to the waste accumulating in the upper, or loose stool or diarrhea due to failure of the nutrients to be sent up.

4. The Large Intestine

The Large Intestine is in the abdomen, with its upper part connecting with the Small Intestine through the blocking gate and its lower part being the anus. The main function of the Large Intestine is to transport and discharge the wastes.

The Large Intestine absorbs the surplus water in the food residues received from the Small Intestine and then turns them into faeces to be discharged through the anus. This function is also a manifestation of the functions of the Stomach in descending turbid and is closely related to the descending effect of the Lung and the sufficiency or Deficiency of the Body Fluid. In the case of sufficiency of Body Fluid, the dispersing and descending effect of the Lung being normally conducted and the Stomach Qi going downwards, the Large Intestine will transform and discharge the waste normally and thus faeces can be discharged regularly and timely. If the Body Fluid is deficient, constipation may occur due to Dryness of the Large Intestine. If the Stomach Qi or the Lung Qi flows upward adversely, constipation due to accumulation of dry stools in the Large Intestine will appear. Conversely, failure of the Large Intestine to transform and discharge will cause upward adversely flow of the Stomach Qi or the Lung Qi, leading to diseases. Besides, the steaming effect of the Kidney is also concerned with the functional activities of the Large Intestine, so there is the saying that the Kidney dominates urination and defecation.

5. The Bladder

The Bladder is located in the center of the lower abdomen, which functions to store urine. As it communicates with the Kidney directly, and the channels of the Kidney and Bladder pertain to and connect with these two organs respectively, the Kidney and Bladder have an interior-exterior relationship. The main functions of the Bladder are to store and discharge urine.

During the process of water metabolism, the water is distributed to the whole body through the effects of the Lung, the Spleen, the Kidney, the Triple Jiao, the Small Intestine and the Large Intestine in order to perform its nourishing and moistening effect. The metabolized water is sent to the Kidney to be turned into urine through the steaming effect of the Kidney and then sent to the Bladder. When the urine retains in the Bladder to certain degree, it is discharged out of the body timely. The storing and discharging effect of the Bladder is completely dependent upon the Kidney's steaming effect. The so-called steaming effect of the Bladder is in fact a part of the steaming effect of the Kidney. If the Kidney Qi is sufficient, the steaming effect of Bladder will be normal, thus the Bladder can open and close regularly to discharge urine. If the Kidney Qi is deficient, the steaming effect will be disturbed, so the Bladder fails to open and close regularly, leading to difficult urination, dribbling of urine, or even retention of urine, or enuresis or even incontinence of urine. If Damp Heat accumulates in Bladder, disturbance of urination will also follow, which is manifested as frequent, urgent and painful urination, hematuria or urolithiasis.

74

6. The Triple Jiao

The Triple Jiao is a collective name for the upper, the lower and the Middle Jiao. As this organ is not so clearly explained in *Huang Di Nei Jing* (The Yellow Emperor's Internal Classics) and it was said to be an organ with its name but without its entity, plenty of controversials arose in the later generations. The focus of the controversials lies in that whether it has a fixed position or entity. At present, some scholars believe that the Triple Jiao is a great Fu organ distributed in the thoracic and abdominal cavities, existing out of the Zang Fu organs and within the trunk, thus it includes all the Zang Fu organs. As it is the greatest organ in the body, it is also known as a solitary organ. However, doctors through ages all believed that the main functions of the Triple Jiao were that it dominates distribution of all the Qi of the body and serves as the passageway of water metabolism.

(1) The main functions of the Triple Jiao:

① Dominating distribution of Qi and the movement and activities of Qi of the whole body: The Triple Jiao is the passageway of the ascending, descending, out-going and entering of Qi and the place where the activities of Qi take place. The primordial Qi, which is the most basic Qi and comes from the Kidney, depends on the Triple Jiao to be distributed to the whole body, thus there is the saying that the Triple Jiao distributes primordial Qi or that the Triple Jiao is where the primordial Qi is to be distributed. All the Qi of the body are distributed to the Five Zang organs and the Six Fu organs through the Triple Jiao to support the life activities. For this reason, it was believed in *Zhong Zang Jing* (A Secret Classics) that the Triple Jiao controls Qi of the Five Zang organs and the Six Fu organs, the defensive Qi and the nutritive Qi, the Qi of the meridians and the Qi of the upper, lower, left and right parts of the body.

② Being the passageway of water flow: The Triple Jiao has the effect of dredging the water metabolism and allowing water to flow through it, so it is the passageway of the ascending, descending, out-going and entering of water in the body. The water metabolism in the whole body is carried out by the Lung, the Spleen and the

Stomach, the intestines, the Bladder and the Kidneys, but it takes the Triple Jiao as its passageway at any rate so that it can be normally distributed. If the Triple Jiao is not smooth, the Lung, the Spleen and the Kidney will not be able to perform their physiological effect in water metabolism. So the effect of the Triple Jiao in coordinating and balancing the water metabolism is known as the steaming effect of the Triple Jiao.

The effect of the Triple Jiao in allowing flow of Qi is closely related to the effect of the Triple Jiao as the passageway of water. This is because that flow of water depends on movements of Qi, and Qi is attached to Blood and Body Fluid to flow. All of these substances take the Triple Jiao as the passageway, therefore, the two functions mentioned above are in fact the two sides of one coin.

(2) Classification of the Triple Jiao and their different physiological functions:

① The Upper Jiao: Usually the Upper Jiao refers to the thorax above the diaphragm which includes the Heart, the Lung and the head and face. Some scholars also ascribe the upper limbs as a part of the Upper Jiao. The Upper Jiao has the function of dispersing and distributing, by which the nutritive substances, Qi, Blood and Body Fluid, are distributed to the whole body to warm and nourish Zang Fu organs, limbs and orifices. So, the function of the Upper Jiao was summarized as a sprayer in *Ling Shu* (The Miraculous Pivot), and based on this, it is suggested in *Wen Bing Tiao Bian* (Analysis of Treatment of Epidemic Febrile Diseases) that drugs with light weight should be adopted in treatment of diseases in the Upper Jiao.

② The Middle Jiao: This refers to the abdomen below the diaphragm and above the umbilicus, mainly including the Spleen and Stomach. The main functions of the Middle Jiao are to ripen food, steam the food essence and produce Qi, Blood and Body Fluid, so it is described as a big tun of distillation in *Ling Shu* (The Miraculous Pivot), and in *Wen Bing Tiao Bian* (Analysis of Treatment of Epidemic Febrile Diseases), it is suggested that drugs with a moderate weight should be employed in treating diseases of the Middle Jiao.

According to the anatomical position, the Liver is situated in the

Middle Jiao. However, in the theory related to epidemic febrile disease in the later generations, Triple Jiao was extended to be a principle for Syndrome identification of epidemic febrile diseases, in which Liver disorders seen in the later stage of epidemic febrile diseases were ascribed to those of the Lower Jiao. In clinical Syndrome identifications today, the Liver is usually regarded as an organ in the Lower Jiao.

③ The Lower Jiao: This indicates the area and the organs below the Stomach or the umbilicus, including the Liver, the Kidney, the Small Intestine, the Large Intestine, the Bladder and the reproductive organs in both male and female. Its main functions are to transport the waste of food and discharge faeces and urine. So, it is described as a ditch of the body in *Ling Shu* (The Miraculous Pivot). Doctors in the later ages have developed the viscera-state theory and attributed the essence and Blood of the Liver and Kidney, Mingmen and the primordial Qi to the Lower Jiao, thus entended the physiological functions of the Lower Jiao. In *Wen Bing Tiao Bian* (Analysis of Treatment of Epidemic Febrile Diseases), it is suggested diseases of the Lower Jiao should be treated with the drugs heavy in nature.

As for the connections between the functions of the Triple Jiao and those of the Zang Fu organs, the function of the Upper Jiao is correspondent to that of the Heart and the Lung; that of the Middle Jiao to that of the Spleen and the Stomach, and that of the Lower Jiao to that of the Liver, the Kidney, the Small Intestine, the Large Intestine, and the Bladder.

The Extraordinary Fu Organs

The extraordinary Fu organs include six organs, the brain, the marrow, the bone, the vessel, the Gallbladder and the uterus. Similar to the Six Fu organs, they are hollow in shape, and similar to the Five Zang organs, they store essence instead of discharging residues of food. Apart from the Gallbladder, the other five organs have not the interior-exterior relationship and usually they are not ascribed to the Five Elements. This makes another difference between the extraordinary Fu organs and the Five Zang organs or the Six Fu organs.

Since the physiology of the vessel, the marrow, the bone and the Gallbladder have been discussed before in this book, they are omitted here.

1. The brain

The brain, located in the cranial cavity, is formed by convergence of marrow, so it is also known as the sea of marrow. In *Da Huo Lun* (A Discussion on Dizziness) of *Ling Shu* (The Miraculous Pivot), detailed discussions on the relations between the brain and the eyes can be read. Based on the descriptions by the ancient doctors, the functions of the brain can be generalized as two aspects. The first aspect is that the brain dominates mental activity, especially the memory, which means that the brain can think about, judge and memorize the external stimuli. When the sea marrow is sufficient, one will be quick at thinking and response and has a strong memory. If the brain is deficient, there will be dizziness, forgetfulness, slow response and poor intelligence. The second is that the brain controls the sensory organs, which means that such sensory organs as the ear, the eye, the mouth, the nose and the tongue all perform their visual, auditory, smelling and tasting functions and the speeching functions under the control of the brain. Thus, when the brain is sufficient, the vision, hearing, smelling and tasting will be good and one's speech will be fluent. If the brain is deficient, disturbance of the visual ability, the auditory ability, the smelling and tasting ability as well as that of speech will occur as a result.

It should be pointed out that the physiological function and the pathological changes of the brain are regarded as those of the Heart and then further ascribed to the Five Zang organs. Therefore, diseases of the brain should be analyzed and treated based on the Five Zang organs instead of on the brain merely.

2. The uterus

78

The uterus is located in the lower abdomen behind the Bladder with a shape of upside placed pear. Its main functions are to develop menstruation and feed fetus. The menstruation and pregnancy are a complicated physiological process, which is concerned with three kinds of physiological factors as mentioned below.

(1) The effect of Tiankui: The development of the reproductive organs completely depends on the effect of Tiankui, which is a product of the constant development of the Kidney essence with the function to promote development and maturity of the sexual glands. Under the action of Tiankui, menstruation occurs following the full development of the reproductive organs in female, which lays the basis for pregnancy. When one reaches the senile age, Tiankui is gradually reduced due to decline of the Kidney essence, so one reaches the menopause period and loses the reproductive ability. Therefore, occurrence and disappearance of Tiankui and the vicissitude of the Kidney essence are the preconditions for the occurrence of menstruation, and serve as the main reason for the maturity and degeneration of the reproductive organs.

(2) The effect of the Chong and Ren Channels: Both the Chong and Ren Channels originate from the uterus. The Chong Channel travels together with the Kidney channel and communicates with the Yangming channel, so it can regulate Qi and Blood in the twelve regular channels and is known as the sea of the twelve regular channels or the sea of Blood. The Ren Channel, meeting with the three Yin channels of feet in the lower abdomen, can regulate the Qi and Blood in all the Yin channels of the human body, so it is also called the sea of Yin channels. When Qi and Blood in the twelve regular channels are adequate, they can enter the Chong and Ren Channels and then to the uterus through the regulation of the Chong and Ren Channels to support menstruation. Tiankui influences the functional states of the Chong and Ren channels. In one's childhood, Tiankui, due to inadequate filling of the essence Qi in the Kidney, is not produced in the body, as a result, Qi and Blood cannot flow in the Ren Channel and are insufficient in the Chong Channel, and thus no menstruation occurs. At the age of puberty, as a result of adequate

filling of the essence Qi in the Kidney, is fully formed in the body, so that Qi and Blood can flow in the Ren Channel, they are sufficient in the Chong Channel and menstruation occurs periodically. When one reaches her senile age, Tiankui declines gradually, so Qi and Blood in the Chong and Ren Channels become less and less and thus she enters the menopause period. Clinically, disturbance of the Chong and Ren Channels may lead to irregular menstruation or even sterility.

(3) The effect of the Heart, the Liver and the Spleen: Both the menstruation and the feeding of fetus depend on nourishment of Qi and Blood. As the Heart dominates Blood, the Liver stores Blood, and the Spleen serves as the source for the generation of Qi and Blood, menstruation and feeding of fetus are closely related to the functional states of these three organs. In the case of failure of the Liver to store Blood or failure of the Spleen to keep Blood flowing within vessels, menorrahge with a long menstrual period and a short interval between two menstruations, or even metrostaxis and metrorrahgia will occur. If the Spleen fails to generate enough Qi and Blood to support the menstruation, there is hypomenorrhea with a long interval or even amenorrhea. Irregular menstruation may also be caused by emotional injury as a result of the impairment of the Heart spirit or failure of the Liver to perform its dispersing and discharging effect.

Connections among Zang Fu Organs

Man is an organic unity composed of a number of Zang Fu organs, channels and tissues. The functional activities of each of the Zang Fu organ and tissues are not isolated, instead, they are a part of the activities of the body as a unity. These organs and tissues restrict each other, depend on each other and supplement each other in the unity, and through the connections of the meridians, they transmit information to each other. In addition, Qi, Blood and Body Fluid flowing over the whole body also contribute to the coordination and unity of human body.

1. Connections among the Five Zang organs

In the ancient times, the relations between Zang organs were usually illustrated in accordance with the generating, restricting, encroaching and violating relations among the Five Elements. Observation and studies in the later generations showed that the relations in the Five Elements cannot reflect the relations among Zang organs completely and precisely. Therefore, the relations of Zang organs are mostly explained on the basis of the different functions of the Zang organs.

The Heart dominates Blood and its flow, while the Lung dominates Qi and respiration, so the relations between the Heart and the Lung are in fact the relations between the Heart's function of controlling Blood and the Lung's function of dominating Qi, and the relations between the Heart's function of promoting flow of Blood and the Lung's function of dominating respiration. The relations between the Heart's function of controlling Blood and the Lung's function of dominating Qi, are, to be more exactly, the relations of mutual dependence and mutual assistance between Qi and Blood. On the one hand, the Lung, which dominates dispersing and descending and meets with all the Blood vessels, can assist the Heart in promoting the Blood flow; on the other hand, normal Blood circulation serves as a prerequisite for the maintenance of the Lung's respiration. Therefore, they often influence each other in pathology.

The Heart has a close relationship with the Spleen. The Heart dominates Blood, while the Spleen can keep Blood flowing within vessels and is where Blood is generated, so the relations between the Heart and the Spleen mainly exist in the generation and circulation of Blood. Pathologically, diseases of the two organs also influence each other, causing such diseases as Deficiency of both the Heart and the Kidney.

The relations between the Liver and the Heart mainly lie in the flow of Blood. The Heart dominates Blood because the Heart Qi is the motive force for Blood flow, while the Liver stores Blood which depends on the normal performance of the Heart's function in moving Blood. Besides, the Heart dominates spirit, while the Liver dominates dispersing and discharging. Although the spirit, thinking and consciousness are governed by the Heart, they are also closely related to the Liver's dispersing and discharging effect.

The relations between the Heart and the Kidney are usually explained according to the ascending and descending movement of Yin and Yang or water and fire. The Heart, pertaining to fire in Five Elements, is located in the upper and is of Yang nature; while the Kidney, pertaining to water in Five Elements, is located in the lower and is of Yin nature. Theoretically, it is believed that the Heart Fire must go down to warm the Kidney and the Kidney water must go up to nourish the Heart so that the physiological functions of these two organs can be harmonious. This is known as coordination between the Heart and the Kidney or between water and fire. When this relation is disturbed, incoordination between the Heart and the Kidney or between the water and fire will ensue. In addition, Yin and Yang of the Heart and the Kidney also have close relationships, so they influence each other in pathological conditions.

Formation of Qi and distribution and discharge of Body Fluid concern both the Lung and the Spleen. Formation of Qi mainly depends on the Lung's respiration and the Spleen's transforming and transporting function, and the distribution and discharge of water are mainly carried out by the Lung's dispersing and descending effect, the Lung's effect of regulating water metabolism and the Spleen's transforming, transporting and distributing effect. So influence of disease of these two organs is mainly reflected as inadequate production of Qi and disturbance of water metabolism. This is why the Spleen is called the source to generate Phlegm and the Lung is where the Phlegm accumulates.

The relations between the Liver and the Lung are mainly manifested in their coordinative functions in regulating movement of Qi. The Lung functions downwards, while the Liver functions upwards, so coordination between them is an important link in maintaining the free flow of Qi of the whole body. The Syndrome of Liver Fire attacking the Lung is just an example of disturbance of the relations between these two organs that is commonly seen in clinic.

The relations between the Lung and the Kidney are mainly reflected on the water metabolism and the respiration. The Kidney is the organ dominating water metabolism, while the Lung is the upper source of water. So the dispersing and descending effects of the Lung in regulating water metabolism depend on the steaming effect of the Kidney Qi. Similarly the effect of the Kidney in dominating water metabolism requires assistance of the Lung's dispersing and descending effect. The Lung dominates exhalation while the Kidney dominates inhalation, so the Lung's respiration requires the assistance of the effect of the Kidney in receiving air. Therefore, there is the saying that the Lung is the organ dominating respiration while the Kidney is the root of respiration. Moreover, Yin Fluids of the two organs nourish each other. For these reasons, mutual influence of diseases of these two organs are often manifested in the water metabolism, respiration and Yin Fluids.

The dispersing and discharging effect of the Liver and the transforming and transporting effect of the Spleen influence each other, which is the main manifestations of the relations between the Liver and the Spleen. In addition, the Liver is also closely related to the Spleen in the formation, storage and flow of Blood. Pathologically, Liver disease may be transmitted to the Spleen or vice versa, and diseases of the two organs often influence each other.

The Liver has a very close relationship with the Kidney, hence there is the saying that the Liver and the Kidney are from the same source. The Liver stores Blood, and the Kidney stores essence. Generation of Blood depends on the steaming effect of the essence Qi of the Kidney, while vicissitude of the essence Qi in the Kidney is determined by the nourishment of Blood. As essence may transform into Blood and vice versa, it is said that the essence and Blood have the same source. Pathologically, diseases of the essence and Blood influence each other. Besides, there exists the mutual restriction and mutual assistance between the Liver's dispersing and discharging effect and the Kidney's storing effect in female's menstruation and male's emission. And as the Liver and the Kidney are from the same source, they also have a close relationship in their Yin and Yang and diseases of them may influence each other.

Physiologically, the relations between the Spleen and the Kidney are in fact the relations between the basis of the congenital constitution and the basis of the acquired constitution. The Spleen is the basis of the acquired constitution, while the Kidney is the basis of the congenital constitution. On one hand, the transforming and transporting effect of the Spleen must be supported by the warming effect of the Kidney Yang, so there is the saying that the Spleen Yang takes the Kidney Yang as its basis. On the other hand, essence Qi stored in the Kidney depends on the nourishment and supplement of the food essence produced by the transforming and transporting effect of the Spleen for its sufficiency and maturity.

2. Connections among the Six Fu organs

The Six Fu organs take transforming and transporting foodstuff as their common physiological functions, so relations among them are mainly embodied in their harmonious connections in digestion, absorption and excretion of the foodstuff.

Entering the Stomach, food is ripened and primarily digested by the Stomach, then it is sent to the Small Intestine to be further digested through the separating effect of the Small Intestine. Following that, the clear part is turned into nutrients through the Spleen's transforming and transporting function to nourish the whole body, while the liquid part of the turbid food seeps into the Bladder and the food residue is sent to the Large Intestine. The liquid entering the Bladder is then transformed into urine through activities of Qi to be discharged timely; while the food residues entering the Large Intestine is conducted and dried to be faeces to be discharged through the anus. In the process of the digestion, absorption, and discharge of food and water, the bile, which can assist in digestion, and the Triple Jiao, which is the passageway of water and food, also play a very important role. The steaming effect of the Triple Jiao, in particular, promotes and supports the transforming and transporting process of food to ensure their normal performance.

Diseases of the Six Fu organs influence each other. Besides, it should be pointed out that disturbance of the Six Fu organs may be either excessive or deficient in nature, although they generally function well when the digestive tract is kept unblocked. So, careful identification and analysis are necessary in the clinic , and over emphasis on the use of the purgatives should be avoided.

3. Connections between the Five Zang organs and the Six Fu organs

The relations between the Five Zang organs and the Six Fu organs can be described as the interior-exterior relationships between Yin and Yang. The Zang organs belong to Yin and are located in the interior, while the Fu organs belong to Yang and are located relatively in the exterior. One Zang organ and one Fu organ, which belong to Yin and Yang, interior and exterior respectively, pair each other to form their close connection through the pertaining-connecting relations between the channels of these two organs. There are five pairs in number, the Heart is interior-exteriorly related to the Small Intestine, the Lung to the Large Intestine, the Spleen to the Stomach, the Liver to the Gallbladder and the Kidney to the Bladder.

Owing to the pertaining-connecting of the their channels, the Heart and the Small Intestine are interior-exteriorly related. The Heart channel pertains to the Heart and connects with the Small Intestine, while the Small Intestine channel pertains to the Small Intestine and connects with the Heart. Pathologically, excessive Heart Fire may be transmitted to the Small Intestine, while Heat in the Small Intestine may go upwards to the Heart along the channels.

The Lung and the Large Intestine are interior-exteriorly related to each other due to pertaining and connecting of their channels. Descending of the Lung Qi can help the Large Intestine to perform its transporting function. On the other hand, normal performance of the transporting effect of the Large Intestine can assist the descending of the Lung Qi. Pathologically, obstruction of the intestine due to excessive Heat in the Large Intestine may obstruct the descending of the Lung Qi, while failure of the Lung Qi to descend may influence the transporting function of the Large Intestine, leading to disorders of defecation.

The Stomach and the Spleen, due to the pertaining-connecting relationships of their channels, are interior-exteriorly related to each other. The Stomach dominates reception of food, while the Spleen dominates transformation and transportation of food. Besides, the Spleen functions upwards, while the Stomach, downwards. So, the functional activities of the Stomach and the Spleen are both supplementary to each other and opposite to each other. Food essence can be distributed normally when the Spleen Qi goes upwards, while the food and its residues can be sent down properly when the Stomach Qi goes downwards. Furthermore, the Stomach likes moistening and is disgusted at Dryness, while the Spleen, likes Dryness and is disgusted at Dampness. Therefore, the food can be transformed and transported only when the Dryness of the Stomach and the Dampness of the Spleen, or the Yang of the Stomach and the Yin of the Spleen, assist each other. Pathologically, disturbance of the transforming and transporting effect of the Spleen due to attack of Dampness will cause inability of the clear Qi (nutrient) to be sent up and failure of the Stomach Qi to perform its receiving effect or go downwards. Conversely, failure of the Stomach Qi may disturb the ascending of the Spleen Qi and the transforming and transporting function of the Spleen.

The Gallbladder is attached to the Liver and their channels pertain to or connect with each other, so the Liver is interior-exteriorly related to the Gallbladder. The bile comes from the residue part of the Liver essence and its secretion and discharge depend on the dispersing and discharging effect of the Liver. However, if the bile is not discharged smoothly, the dispersing and discharging effect of the Liver may also be disturbed. Pathologically, disease often occurs in both the Liver and Gallbladder as a result of the Liver diseases affecting the GallBladder or vice versa.

The Kidney and the Bladder are interior-exteriorly related to each

86

other because their channels pertain to and connect with them re-spectively. The function of the Bladder, storing and discharging urine, is determined by the steaming effect of the Kidney. So, when the Kidney Qi is sufficient and the Kidney can control the opening and closing movement of the Bladder, water metabolism will be nor-mal. On the contrary, failure of the Kidney to control the opening and closing of the Bladder, as a result of Deficiency of the Kidney Qi, will cause disturbance of urination.

Qi, Blood
and Body Fluid

*Q*i, Blood and Body Fluid are all the basic substances constituting the human body and serve as the material basis for
the physiological functions of the Zang Fu organs and tissues.

Qi is a vigorous substance flowing constantly. Blood is basically
the same with the Blood in Western medicine in its appearance, and
the Body Fluid is a general term for all the normal fluids of the human body. In accordance with their relative properties, Qi, which
has the warming and propelling function, belongs to Yang, and
Blood and Body Fluid, which function to nourish and moisten the
human body, belong to Yin.

Qi, Blood and Body Fluid are the material basis of the functional
activities of Zang Fu organs, channels and tissues and the also products of these activities. So, there exist a mutual supplementing and
a cause-result relationship between the Qi, Blood and Body Fluid
and the Zang Fu organs and channels in both physiology and pathology.

In addition, essence is also a basic substance constituting the human body. It has two meanings. In a broad sense, it refers to all the
refined substances or the nutritive substances of the human body,

including Qi, Blood, Body Fluid and other nutritive substances; in a narrow sense, it refers to the congenital essence stored in the Kidney, which has been discussed before.

Qi

1. Concept of Qi

Qi comes from the understanding of the ancient Chinese on the natural phenomena. In Chinese ancient philosophy, Qi is regarded as the most basic substance constituting the world. In the theoretical system of TCM, Qi refers to a refined vigorous substance that is in constant motion. It is both a basic substance constituting the human body and a basic substance maintaining life activities of the human body.

Qi of the human body may exist in two forms: the congealed Qi such as the Zang organ, the Fu organ, the body tissues, the orifices, essence, Blood and Body Fluid, and the diffusive Qi which is invisible, such as the genuine Qi, the pectorial Qi, the defensive Qi and the nutritive Qi. In accordance with the traditional understanding of TCM through ages, Qi here mainly refers to the latter.

Movement of Qi is the most basic movement of the life activities. In order to maintain the life, one must absorb the essence Qi from nature constantly. All the movements and activities of the human body depend on the propelling effect of Qi. Therefore, the life activities are in fact the motions and changes of Qi of the human body. If Qi of the body is unable to move and change, life activities will end. This is why Qi is considered the most basic substance constituting the human body.

2. Formation of Qi

Qi of the human body is formed by the congenital Qi inherited from parents, the essence Qi contained in food and the fresh air existing in nature through the combined action of the Lung, the Spleen, the Stomach and the Kidney.

The congenital Qi can only perform its physiological effect when the Kidney can store essence. The essence contained in food depends on the transforming and transporting function of the Spleen and Stomach to be absorbed. And the fresh air existing in nature depends on the respiratory effect of the Lung for its inhalation. For this reason, formation of Qi is closely related to the functional states of the Kidney, the Spleen, the Stomach and the Lung, as well as the congenital constitution, the food nutrition and the natural environments. When the functional activities of the Kidney, the Spleen, the Stomach and the Lung are kept normal and balanced, Qi of the human body can be kept sufficient. On the contrary, if any of the functional activities of these organs or the harmony between these activities is disturbed, Qi cannot be formed properly or cannot perform its physiological effect normally, leading to such pathological changes as Deficiency of Qi.

In the process of the generation of Qi, the transforming and transporting effect of the Spleen and the Stomach plays a very important role. After his birth, man completely depends on nourishment of the nutrients contained in food for maintaining his life activities, and the absorption of the nutrients completely depends on the receiving and the transforming and transporting effects of the Spleen and the Stomach so that the food can be digested, absorbed and turned into food essence. The congenital essence also depends on the supplement of the food essence so that it can give full play of its physiological effect. Therefore it is said in *Wu Wei* (Five Tastes) in *Ling Shu* (The Miraculous Pivot) that "If one doesn't eat for half a day, his Qi will become weak, while if he doesn't eat for a day, he will has less Qi. "

3. Physiological functions of Qi

Qi has a number of important physiological functions in the human body, which can be generalized as the following five kinds:

(1) Propelling effect: Qi is a vigorous substance which can propel and initiate the growth and development of the human body, the functional activities of Zang Fu organs, the formation and circulation of Blood, and the generation, distribution and discharge of

90

Body Fluid. When Qi is deficient or its propelling and initiating effect declines, there will be early aging as a result of disturbance of the growth and development of the human body, or functional decline of the Zang Fu organs or channels, or Blood Deficiency, disturbance of Blood flow and water retention as a result of inadequate production and sluggish flow of Blood and Body Fluid.

(2) Warming effect: This means that Qi is the source of the heat required by the body. The body temperature is kept constant by the warming effect of Qi, the functional activities of Zang Fu organs and meridians also depend on the warming effect of Qi for their normal performance. In addition, such liquid substances as Blood and Body Fluid cannot circulate or flow normally unless they are warmed by Qi. So there is a saying that Blood will flow freely in the case of being warmed and will flow slowly or stagnate if it is cooled. When the warming effect of Qi declines, such cold manifestations as aversion to cold, cold limbs, desire for warmth, reduce of body temperature or slow flow of Blood and Body Fluid will ensue. If Qi stagnates and turns into Heat for some reasons, it will cause aversion to heat, desire for cold or fever as a result of strengthening of its warming effect.

(3) Defending effect: The defending effect of the human body is a combined effect of various organs, tissues and substances of the human body such as Qi, Blood, Body Fluid, Zang Fu organs and meridians. Of these organs, tissues and substances, the effect of Qi is the most important, which mainly lies in that Qi can protect the skin and muscles of the human body from invasion of pathogenic factors. If the defending effect of Qi declines, the resistant ability of the human body will be lowered, as a result, diseases are likely to occur. This is what is said in *Ping Re Bing Lun* (Comments on Febrile Disease) in *Su Wen* (The Plain Questions), "Where the pathogens attack, where Qi is deficient. "

(4) Controlling effect: This means that Qi can prevent useless loss of such liquid substances as Blood and Body Fluid. It is mainly manifested as the following aspects: keeping Blood flowing within vessels to prevent extravasation, and controlling the secretion and

91

discharge of such liquids as sweat, urine, saliva, gastric juice, intestinal juice and sperm to prevent their excessive discharge. When this effect of Qi is weakened, massive loss of the liquid substances will follow as a consequence. For example, failure of Qi to control Blood may cause various kinds of bleedings; failure of Qi to control Body Fluid may lead to spontaneous sweating, profuse urine or incontinence of urine, dribbling, vomiting watery fluid, diarrhea, or incontinence of defecation; and inability of Qi to consolidate emission may cause nocturnal emission, spermatorrhea or premature ejaculation.

The controlling effect and the propelling effect of Qi are both opposite to each other and supplementary to each other. The harmonious performance of these two different effects ensures the normal regulation and control of the flow, secretion and discharge of the liquid substances of the human body, which serves as an important link in maintenance of the normal Blood circulation and water metabolism.

(5) Steaming effect: Changes caused by movement of Qi are called *Qi Hua* in TCM, which, to be more precise, indicates the metabolism of essence, Qi, Blood and Body Fluid in the human body and their mutual transformation. For example, formation of Qi, Blood and Body Fluid depends on the food essence transformed from food; the Body Fluid, after being metabolized, will turn into sweat and urine; and the residue part of food, after being digested and absorbed, will transform into the wastes. All these changes are the signs of the steaming effect of Qi. If Qi fails to steam, various kinds of disturbance of metabolism will present as a result of abnormality of the metabolism of these substances, the digestion and absorption of food and the discharge of sweat, urine and faeces. Therefore, the process of Qi performing its steaming effect is just a process of transformation of the substances and energy of the human body.

4. Movement of Qi and its basic forms

Qi of the human body is a vigorous substance in constant motion. It flows and exists in all the organs and tissues of the body such as the Zang Fu organs and meridians, so that it can propel and initiate various kinds of life activities.

Movement of Qi is also known as mechanism of Qi. Although Qi may move in many different ways, these movements can be generalized theoretically into four basic types: ascending, descending, outgoing and entering, which are the basis of the life activities and exist throughout one's whole life. Once the movements of Qi end, life activities will find their terminals.

On the one hand, the ascending, descending, out-going and entering movements of Qi propel and initiate the physiological activities of the human body; on the other hand, they are embodied concretely in the physiological activities of the Zang Fu organs and meridians. All the organs and tissues of the human body, including the Zang Fu organs and meridians, are where the Qi's ascending, descending outgoing and entering movements take place. For example, in the process of respiration dominated by the Lung, exhalation is a movement of ascending; inhalation is a movement of descending; dispersing effect of the Lung is a process of ascending, and the purifying and descending effect of the Lung is a sign of descending movement of Qi. All the life activities of the human body are in fact the concrete manifestations of the ascending, descending, outgoing and entering movements of Qi.

The ascending movement and the descending movements of Qi is a unity of opposite, and this is also true to the outgoing and entering movements of Qi. However, in a local area, it is not that every physiological function can be generalized as these four aspects, instead, it may be only a sign of one of the four types of movement of Qi. For example, the Liver and the Spleen dominate ascending, while the Lung and the Stomach dominate descending. But as a whole, the ascending and descending, the outgoing and entering of Qi in the whole body must be kept in harmony and balance in order to maintain the normal life activities of the human body. Therefore, the ascending, descending, outgoing and entering movements of Qi play an important role in coordinating and balancing the different physiological functions of the human body.

The harmonious balance among the ascending, descending, outgoing and entering movements of Qi is known as and harmony of Qi's movements; while disturbance of the harmonious balance is called disturbance of Qi's movements. Disturbance of Qi's movements are various, but stagnation of Qi, upward adverse flow of Qi, sinking of Qi, escape of Qi and obstruction of Qi are commonly encountered in the clinic.

5. Distribution and classification of Qi

Qi of the human body flows throughout the whole body. As the components, distributions and functions of Qi are different, Qi has different names. The most important Qi of the body are as follows:

(1) The Primordial Qi: Also known as genuine Qi or true Qi, the primordial Qi is the most basic and the most important Qi of the human body. It is regarded as the primordial motive force of the life activities of the human body.

① Components and distribution of the primordial Qi: The primordial Qi mainly comes from the essence Qi stored in the Kidney, which originally comes from the congenital essence inherited from parents and further supplemented by the food essence produced by the Spleen. Therefore, vicissitude of the primordial Qi is closely related to both the congenital constitution and the transforming and transporting effect of the Spleen and the Stomach.

The primordial Qi is distributed to the whole body through Triple Jiao to perform its effect in every part of the body.

② Main functions of the primordial Qi. Being the primordial motive force of the life activities of the human body and the basic substance maintaining the life activities, the primordial Qi can promote the growth and development of the human body, and warm and initiate the physiological functions of the Zang Fu organs and tissues. Therefore, when the primordial Qi is replete, the functional activities of the Zang Fu organs and meridians will be strong, thus one has a strong constitution and is less affected by disease. If, due to congenital defect, improper feeding after birth or consumption in chronic disease, the primordial Qi is deficient, various kinds of diseases will follow.

(2) The pectoral Qi: The pectoral Qi is one accumulating in the

thorax. Where the pectoral Qi is accumulated in the thorax is also called "the sea of Qi" or *Shan Zhong*.

① Components and distribution of the pectoral Qi: The pectoral Qi comes from combination of the fresh air inhaled by the Lung from nature and the food essence transformed and transported by the Spleen from foodstuff. Therefore, vicissitude of the pectoral Qi is directly concerned with both the respiratory function of the Lung and the transforming and transporting function of the Spleen.

The pectoral Qi accumulating in the thorax is distributed up to the throat and down to the Heart vessels and the groin where it is further sent to all the whole body under the action of the dispersing effect of the Lung.

② Main functions of the pectoral Qi: The pectoral Qi has two functions: travelling in the respiratory tract to promote respiration and going through the Heart vessels to promote flow of Qi and Blood. The former function is related to speech, voice and respiration, while the latter is concerned with the flow of Qi and Blood, coldness or warmth of the limbs and their activities, such sensory functions as seeing and hearing, strength of the Heart beats and the Heart rhythm.

(3) The nutritive Qi: The nutritive Qi is one that flows together with Blood in the vessels. As it is rich in nutrients, it is so named; and as it has a very close relationship with Blood and is difficult to be clearly differentiated from Blood, it is often called together with Blood as *Ying Xue* (nutritive Qi and Blood). Besides, as it belongs to Yin compared with the defensive Qi, it is also named *Ying Yin* (nutritive Yin).

① Components and distribution of the nutritive Qi: The nutritive Qi is mainly derived from the refined part of the food essence transformed and transported by the Spleen. Distributed circularly and endlessly in the vessels and as a component part of Blood, it flows in the vessels together with Blood to Zang Fu organs internally and limbs externally.

② Main functions of the nutritive Qi: The nutritive Qi has two main functions: generating Blood, which means that the nutritive Qi

95

can absorb Body Fluid from the foodstuff and then induce it into vessels to generate Blood; and nourishing the whole body, which means that all the Five Zang organs, the Six Fu organs, the limbs and all the bones of the body can maintain their normal physiological functions only when they are well nourished by the nutritive Qi.

(4) The defensive Qi: The defensive Qi is one that flows outside vessels. As it belongs to Yang compared with the nutritive Qi, it is also named the defensive Yang.

① Components and distribution of the defensive Qi: The defensive Qi comes from the thick and vigorous part of the food essence, so it is vigorous, smooth, active and swift in flow. Therefore, it is not limited by the vessel and flows outside vessels to the whole body including the Zang Fu organs in the interior and the skin and muscles in the exterior.

② Main functions of the defensive Qi: Functions of the defensive Qi are threefold: firstly, it can protect the skin and muscles from invasion of exogenous pathogenic factors; secondly, it can warm and nourish the Zang Fu organs, muscles and skins; and thirdly, it can control and regulate opening and closing of the striae of muscles and the discharge of sweat to maintain the relative stability of the body temperature.

Both the nutritive Qi and the defensive Qi are derived from the food essence. But the nutritive Qi flows in the vessels, belongs to Yin and functions inwards; while the defensive Qi flows outside the vessels, defends the exterior and belongs to Yang. So they must be kept in harmony in order to maintain the normal opening and closing movements of striae of muscles, the body temperature and the resistant ability of the body against the exogenous pathogens. Otherwise, disharmony between them will cause chills and fever, absence of sweating or profuse sweating, and lowering of the resistant ability of the body against pathogens.

Apart from the four kinds of Qi mentioned above, Qi of the human body also includes such Qi as Qi of Zang Fu organs and Qi of the meridians, which are generally considered to be secondary to the primordial Qi. In other words, when the primordial Qi is distributed to an organ or meridian, it becomes Qi of the organ or the meridian. Qi of the Zang Fu organ or meridian is a part of the primordial Qi, so it is the most basic substance constituting the organ and meridian and serves as the material basis promoting and maintaining the physiological functions of the Zang Fu organs and meridians.

In TCM theory, there are still many things named after Qi. For example, the nutrient absorbed from food is also called food essence or food Qi; causative factor of disease is also termed pathogenic Qi; the physiological function and the resistant ability of the body is called Vital Qi or righteous Qi; the abnormal water in the body is called water Qi; and the four kinds of natures or properties of drugs are named four kinds of Qi, etc. All these Qi are different from the Qi as a basic substance constituting the human body.

Blood

1. Concept of Blood

Blood is a red liquid substance with a strong tonifying and nourishing effect. It is also a basic substance constituting the human body and maintaining the life activities of the human body.

Blood flows in the Blood vessels to the whole body. As the vessel is where the Blood circulates and has the effect of preventing extravasation, it is also named Blood house. Blood can perform its normal physiological functions only when it flows in the vessels. If Blood escapes from the vessels, bleeding will ensue. The extravasated Blood is therefore known as Blood out of vessels.

2. Formation of Blood

Blood is mainly composed of nutritive Qi and Body Fluid, both of which originate from the food essence generated through the Spleen's transforming and transporting effect. Therefore the Spleen is also called the source for production of Qi and Blood. As for the concrete process of the Blood formation, there is no unified understanding in *Huang Di Nei Jing* (The Yellow Emperor's Internal

Classics), although this is mentioned in many paragraphs of the book. Generally speaking, the main material basis of formation of Blood is the combined nutritive Qi and Body Fluid and the vessels are where the Blood is formed. As both the nutritive Qi and Body Fluid are from the food essence, quality of food and the functional states of the Spleen and the Stomach may directly influence the generation of Blood. Long-standing inadequate intake of food or nutrients or disturbance of the functional activities of the Spleen and Stomach can lead to inadequate production of Blood, causing Blood Deficiency.

In addition, there exist the relations of mutual assistance and transformation between the essence and Blood. The essence is stored in the Kidney, while the Blood is stored by the Liver. If the Kidney essence is sufficient, the Liver will be well tonified and the Blood stored in the Liver will be well supplemented. Or the other way round, if the Liver stores enough Blood, the Kidney essence will be well assisted. So there is the saying that both the essence and Blood are derived from the same source.

3. Functions of Blood

Blood has the function of nourishing and moistening the whole body, which is summarized in *Nan Jing* (The Difficult Classics) as "The Blood functions to nourish the body." To be concrete, the functions of Blood include the following three aspects:

(1) Supporting the life activities of the Zang Fu organs, body tissues and nine orifices of the body: Blood, flowing through the vessels endlessly and circularly to the Zang Fu organs internally and the bones, muscles and skins externally, nourishes and moistens these organs and tissues constantly and supports their life activities. When Blood is sufficient, there will be red and lustrous face, lustrous skin and hair, indurated bones and tendons, fine muscles and strong Zang Fu organs. If Blood is inadequate, there will be sallow complexion, withered skin and hair, weakness of bones and tendons, emaciated muscles and fragile Zang Fu organs. So the ancients said that "Blood sufficiency causes the body to be strong, while Blood Deficiency leads to weakness of the body."

98

(2) Supporting the movements and sensory functions of the body: The movements and sensory functions of the body depend on nourishment of Blood. Just as stated in *Wu Zang Sheng Cheng Pian* (Formation of the Five Zang Organs) of *Su Wen* (The Plain Questions): "Because of nourishment of Blood, the eyes can see, the feet can walk, the hands can grasp, and the fingers can pick." Clinically, Blood Deficiency often gives rise to dizziness, vertigo, blurred vision, tinnitus, numbness of limbs without strength, or convulsion or even flaccidity of tendons and bones.

(3) Supporting the mental activities: Blood is the main substance supporting the mental activities. Sufficiency of Qi and Blood and free flow of Blood in the vessels will present being full of vigour, clear mind, strong senses amd flexible movements. On the contrary, weakness of vigour, forgetfulness, dream-disturbed sleep, insomnia and dysphoria, or even dementia, palpitation, delirium and coma may appear as a result of Blood Deficiency, Blood Heat or abnormal circulation of Blood.

4. Circulation of Blood

The Blood circulates in the vessels endlessly to be distributed to the whole body to provide rich nourishment to all the Zang Fu organs and tissues of the body. Blood flow mainly depends on the propelling effect of Qi, also, Blood depends on the controlling effect of Qi to flow within vessels instead of extravasating. Therefore, it is the harmony and balance between the propelling effect and the controlling effect of Qi that maintain the normal flow of Blood. These effects of Qi are carried out by different functions of Zang Fu organs, of which functions of the Heart, the Liver, the Spleen and the Lung are most closely concerned. To be more exact, the Blood flow depends on the propelling of the Heart beats, the propelling and the promoting of the dispersing effect of the Lung where all Blood converges and the dispersing and discharging effect of the Liver; and that the Spleen keeps Blood flowing in vessels and that the Liver stores Blood are both the important factors contributing to control of Blood flow. In addition, the normal flow of Blood also depends on whether the vessels are smooth and whether the temperature of

Blood is normal or not. Therefore, normal flow of Blood is determined not only by the physiological functions of the Heart, but also by whether the functional activities of the Lung, the Spleen and the Liver are harmonious or not. In the case of increase of the factors propelling and promoting Blood flow, or decline of the factors controlling Blood flow, Blood will flow faster than normal or even flows out of vessels. Conversely, in the case of decline of the factors propelling and promoting Blood flow or increase of the factors controlling Blood flow, the Blood will flow slower than normal, leading to Blood Stasis, etc.

Body Fluid

1. Concept of Body Fluid

Body Fluid is a general term for all the normal liquid of the human body. Like Qi and Blood, it is also a basic substance constituting the human body and maintaining the life activities of the human body. It includes the fluids in the Zang Fu organs and tissues, and the normal secretions of the human body such as the gastric juice, intestinal juice, nasal discharge, tear, etc.

Body Fluid, or Jin Ye in Chinese, can be divided into two kinds in accordance with their different natures, functions and distributions: Jin and Ye. Jin refers to the clear part of Body Fluid which is more mobile, mainly distributed to the skin, muscles and orifices and can seep into vessels with moistening as its main function, while Ye refers to the thick part of the Body Fluid which is not so mobile and is mainly infused into the joints, Zang Fu organs, brain and bone marrow with nourishing as its main function. Jin and Ye are often called together because they may transform into each other, but they should be differentiated in the case of impairment of Jin or escape of Ye.

2. Formation, distribution and discharge of Body Fluid

This is a complicated process involving a series of physiological functions of many Zang Fu organs. The Body Fluid is originated from foodstuff, the liquid part of food is gradually digested and absorbed through the receiving and ripening effect of the Stomach and the separating effect of the Small Intestine, then it turns into Body Fluid through the absorption, transformation and transportation of the Spleen. As for its distribution and discharge, it depends on the transporting effect of the Spleen, the dispersing and descending effect of the Lung and the steaming effect of the Kidney to be distributed to the whole body through the Triple Jiao.

The transporting effect of the Spleen in the distribution of Body Fluid is also called the Spleen Qi distributing water essence, which is mainly manifested as two aspects: firstly, it sends the Body Fluid up to the Lung to be further distributed to the Zang Fu organs, body tissues and orifices through the dispersing and descending effect of the Lung; secondly, it can send the Body Fluid directly outwards to the whole body. If the Spleen fails to perform its transforming and transporting effect, the formation and distribution of Body Fluid will be disturbed, hence there goes the saying that all diseases marked by edema or abdominal fullness are caused by disorder of the Spleen.

The Lung regulates water metabolism through its dispersing and descending effect. Receiving the Body Fluid transported from the Spleen, the Lung, on the one hand, sends the Body Fluid outwards and upwards to the upper part and the exterior of the human body through its dispersing effect. On the other hand, it sends the Body Fluid downwards and inwards to the Kidney, the Bladder and other tissues in the lower part of the body through its descending effect. In the case of disturbance of the dispersing and descending effect of the Lung, water will fail to be dredged and thus it will retain to form Phlegm or water retention, or even cause edema in severe cases.

The Kidney plays a leading role in distribution and discharge of Body Fluid. Firstly, the steaming effect of the essence Qi of the Kidney propels the formation, distribution and discharge of the Body Fluid. The effects of the Stomach, and the Small Intestine, the Spleen and the Lung in water metabolism all depend on the steaming effect of the Kidney to be carried out; secondly, the metabolized Body Fluid can be turned into urine through the steaming effect of the Kidney and then infused into Bladder to be discharged; and thirdly, the kidney controls the volume of urine to regulate the balance of water metabolism of the whole body.

The Body Fluid is discharged in the form of urine, sweat, the vapourized water in breathing and water in faeces.

Distribution and discharge of Body Fluid in the whole body can also be generalized as the ascending, descending, outgoing and entering movement of the Body Fluid, which is carried out by the induction of the ascending, descending, outgoing and entering movements of Qi under the action of the steaming effect of the Kidney with the Triple Jiao as its passageway. Balance of the formation, distribution and discharge of the Body Fluid results from the harmonious balance of the functions of Qi and different Zang Fu organs, especially the functions of the Lung, the Spleen and the Kidney. So, disorder of Qi or disorders of Zang Fu organs will influence the formation, distribution and discharge of Body Fluid, destroy balance of the water metabolism, leading to impairment of Jin, escape of Ye or insufficiency of Body Fluid, or water retention in the body such as edema, Dampness and Phlegm.

3. Functions of Body Fluid

The Body Fluid has both moistening and nourishing effects. As it is a liquid substance, it has a strong moistening effect; and as it contains plentiful nutritive substances, it has a strong nourishing effect. Theoretically, Jin should has a stronger moistening effect because it is thinner in quality, while Ye has a stronger nourishing effect because it is thicker. The moistening and nourishing effects of Body Fluid can be seen in many parts of the human body. For example, the Body Fluid distributed to the skin and muscle can moisten and nourish the skin, hair and the muscles; the Body Fluid infused into the orifices can moist, nourish and protect the eyes, nose, mouth, etc., the Body Fluid seeping into Blood vessels can nourish the Blood and allow the vessels to be smooth and supplement Blood;

the Body Fluid flowing to the internal organs and tissues can nourish and moisten these organs and tissues, and that infused into bones can nourish the bone marrow, the spinal marrow and the brain marrow.

Relations between Qi, Blood and Body Fluid

Although Qi, Blood and Body Fluid are different in natures and functions, they all come from the food essence transformed and transported by the Spleen, and they are all the most basic substances constituting the human body and supporting the life activities of the human body. So, there exist the mutual dependence, mutual transformation and mutual assistance relationship among them.

1. Relations between Qi and Blood

Qi is a Yang substance while Blood belongs to Yin. In *Er Shi Er Nan* (The 22th Question) of *Nan Jing* (The Difficult Classics), the different functions of Qi and Blood are summarized as that "Qi mainly has a warming effect while Blood mainly has a nourishing effect." The close relations between Qi and Blood are usually generalized as two aspects: Qi being the commander of Blood and Blood being the mother of Qi.

(1) Qi being the commander of Blood: This is mainly manifested as three aspects:

① Qi being able to generate Blood: This means that formation and production of Blood have close relationships with Qi and its activities. Nutritive Qi and Body Fluid, the main raw materials to form Blood, both come from the food essence transformed and transported by the Spleen and the Stomach; and transformation of food into food essence, transformation of food essence into nutritive Qi and Body Fluid and the final generation of the red Blood all depend on Qi's activities. So it is said that Qi can generate Blood.

103

When Qi is sufficient, it will has a strong effect in generating Blood, while if it is deficient, its function of generating Blood will be poor, which may further cause Blood Deficiency. Therefore, drugs tonifying Qi are often adopted to treat Blood Deficiency in the clinic in order to improve the therapeutic effects.

② Qi being able to move Blood: Blood is a Yin substance, thus it cannot move itself and depends on the propelling of Qi for its flow. Flow of Blood results from the propelling effect of the Heart Qi, the dispersing and distributing effect of the Lung Qi and the dredging and dispersing effect of the Liver. When Qi flows normally, Blood will flow freely; when Qi is deficient, it will not be able to move Blood; and when Qi stagnates, Blood flow will be obstructed. Adverse flow of Qi may also cause adverse flow of Blood. Thus, drugs supplementing Qi, promoting flow of Qi and lowering Qi are often employed in the clinic to treat disorders marked by abnormal Blood flow.

③ Qi being able to control Blood flow: This is a concrete manifestation of the controlling effect of Qi. It is just because of the controlling effect of Qi that Blood flows within vessels instead of out of the vessels. Therefore, decline of Qi's controlling effect due to its Deficiency may lead to various kinds of bleedings, known as failure of Qi to control Blood. When such cases are treated, the therapeutic method, supplementing Qi to control Blood, should be adopted.

(2) Blood being the mother of Qi: This means that Blood carries Qi and provides sufficient nutrients for Qi. As Qi is a vigorous substance, it has a tendency to escape from the human body, so it must be attached to Blood and Body Fluid to perform its normal functions in the human body. If Qi fails to be attached to the Blood, it will lose its basis and float, causing escape of Qi. Besides, the functional activities of Qi also depend on nourishment of the Blood. Any part of the human body, if poorly nourished by Blood, will not be able to perform its functional activities. If Zang Fu organs and tissues cannot perform their physiological functions, Qi cannot be generated. Therefore, Qi Deficiency is likely to occur when Blood is deficient, and massive bleeding may be followed by escape of Qi.

104

2. Relations between Qi and Body Fluid

Qi belongs to Yang while Body Fluid to Yin. So the relations between Qi and Body Fluid are very similar to these between Qi and Blood. That is, the formation, distribution and discharge of Body Fluid fully depend on Qi's movements and the steaming, warming, propelling and controlling effects of Qi; while Qi also depends on carrying of Body Fluid for its existence in the body and its movements.

(1) Effect of Qi on Body Fluid:

① Qi being able to generate Body Fluid: Body Fluid comes from the food and water the human body takes in, and the process of the transformation of food and water into Body Fluid depends on the transforming and transporting effects of the Spleen. Therefore, if the Spleen Qi and the Stomach Qi are sufficient, there will be enough Body Fluid to be generated. On the contrary, in the case of Deficiency of the Spleen Qi and the Stomach Qi, Body Fluid will be inadequately produced, or even impairment of both Qi and Body Fluid will follow as a result.

② Qi being able to move or steam Body Fluid: Distribution and discharge of Body Fluid depend on ascending, descending, outgoing and entering movements of Qi. The Body Fluid is distributed to the whole body to ensure the balance of water metabolism only when the Spleen can send up nutrients and transport fluids, the Lung can disperse and descend fluids and the Kidney can steam fluids. Therefore, disturbance of Qi's movements will certainly cause sluggish distribution and discharge of Body Fluid, and retentions of Body Fluid of varying causes will give rise to disturbance of the ascending, descending, outgoing and entering movements of Qi. As a result of their influence, such pathological changes as water retention, Phlegm, Dampness or even edema due to overflow of water to the skin often result, which should be treated with both the drugs promoting flow of Qi and the drugs eliminating water in the clinic.

③ Qi being able to control discharge of Body Fluid: Qi has the effect of controlling the discharge of Body Fluid to prevent its useless loss. For example, the defensive Qi can consolidate opening and

105

closing of the sweat pores and the Kidney Qi can control the opening and closing of the anus and the Bladder to prevent excessive loss of Body Fluid. If Qi fails to perform its controlling effect, Body Fluid will be discharged excessively, leading to profuse sweating, spontaneous sweating, massive urine or enuresis, etc.

(2) Effect of Body Fluid on Qi: Qi is an invisible substance that is likely to dismiss, so it must be attached to the visible Body Fluid to exist in the body and to be distributed to the whole body, hence there is the saying that Body Fluid carries Qi. When Body Fluid is discharged excessively, Qi will follow the discharge of fluid to dismiss, which is known as escape of Qi following discharge of Body Fluid. For example, profuse sweating, severe vomiting and diarrhea or profuse urine will not only impair the Body Fluid, but also impair Qi, leading to general weakness. This is what is said that Qi in a patient with severe vomiting or diarrhea will certainly be injured.

3. Relations between Blood and Body Fluid

Both Blood and Body Fluid are the liquid substances coming from the same source with similar functions and a mutual transformation relationship, so they have a very close relationship.

Blood and Body Fluid are said to come from the same source because both of them are generated from the food essence produced by the transforming and transporting effects of the Spleen. As for the nature and functions, Blood and Body Fluid are both visible things and still in nature, so they belong to Yin and have the function of moistening and nourishing. Blood circulates in vessels, while Body Fluid may exist in or out of the vessels. When the Body Fluid is infused into the vessels, it combines with nutritive Qi to become the red Blood, while if it goes out of the vessels, it separates from the nutritive Qi to be Body Fluid again.

As a result of their close connections in physiology, disorder of Blood and that of Body Fluid influence each other. For example, when massive loss of Blood occurs, Body Fluid outside of the vessels will enter the vessels to make up the losed Blood, causing such symptoms as thirst, scanty urine, or dry skin. Or the other way round, when Body Fluid is consumed massively, there will not be enough Body Fluid to be infused into the vessels and Body Fluid in the vessels will go out of the vessels to cause emptiness of the vessels and Blood Dryness due to depletion of Body Fluid. For this reason, it is suggested that diaphoretics should be adopted carefully in the case of Blood loss and drugs removing Blood Stasis should be less selected in the case of profuse sweating.

Meridians

*M*eridian theory is a subject dealing with the physiological function and the pathological change of meridians and their connections with Zang Fu organs. It is an important part of the TCM theories.

The meridian theory originated in the long-standing clinical practice of the ancient Chinese, who developed this theory based on their clinical experience in acupuncture and moxibustion, tuina therapy and qigong therapy, etc. as well as the anatomical knowledge at that time. It has a universe guiding significance to all the clinical branches of TCM and serves as the theoretical basis of the acupuncture and moxibustion, tuina and qigong practice. In order to explain completely the physiological functions and the pathological changes of the human body and guide the diagnosis and treatment of diseases, such theories as viscera-state theory, the theory of Qi, Blood and Body Fluid, the theory of etiology and the theory of meridians must be adopted together. Therefore, it is said that one will always make mistakes in diagnosis and treatment of disease if he doesn't know anything about meridians.

Meridians and Components
of the Meridian System

1. Concept of meridian

Meridians, which connect the Zang Fu organs with the limbs, the
upper with the lower, and the exterior with the interior, are the
passageways through which Qi and Blood are distributed to the
whole body. The meridian is a collective term for channels and collaterals. Channels are the main trunks of the meridian system that
travels in the depth of the body along certain route, while the collaterals are the branches of the meridian system, which run in the superficial parts of the body or even emerge in the exterior of the
body. They are distributed vertically and horizontally, linking every
part of the whole body like a net. As a result, all the organs and tissues of the human body, including the Zang Fu organs, orifices, the
skin, the muscles, the tendons and the bones, are linked up with
each other, and the human body is integrated into an organic unity.

2. Components of the meridian system

The meridian system includes two parts, channels and collaterals. They connects with Zang Fu organs interiorly and the tendons
and skins exteriorlly.

Channels can be divided into two kinds, the regular channels and
the extraordinary channels. The regular channels, composed of the
three Yin channels and the three Yang channels of hands and feet,
are twelve in number, so they are called the twelve regular channels. The twelve regular channels are the main passageway in which
Qi and Blood circulate. They have fixed starting points, terminals,
distributing routes in limbs, connecting order, and direct pertaining-
connecting relationships with the Zang Fu organs. The extraordinary channels, including the Du Channel, the Ren Channel, the Dai
Channel, the Chong Channel, the Yinwei Channel, the Yangwei
Channel, the Yinqiao Channel and the Yangqiao Channel, are eight

in number, so they are called the eight extraordinary channels collectively. The eight extraordinary channels function to control and connect the twelve regular meridians and regulate Qi and Blood in the twelve regular meridians. In addition, the channel system also includes the channels branching off from the twelve regular channels, which are collectively known as the twelve branches of the channels. Originating from the four limbs, all these branches run to and travel in the depth of Zang Fu organs in the body cavity, then emerge in the neck or nape where the branches of the Yang channels go back to the channels they branch off and those of the Yin channels enter the Yang channels interior-exteriorly related. The branches of the twelve regular channels function to strengthen connections of the interior-exteriorly related channels and to reach some areas the regular channels do not.

Collaterals are the branches of the channels, which are classified as three groups, the major collaterals, the superficial collaterals and the minute collaterals. The major collaterals are the main part of the collateral system, including the major collaterals of the twelve regular channels, these of the Ren and Du Channels and that of the Spleen, which are collectively called the fifteen major collaterals. The main function of the major collaterals is to strengthen connections of the interior-exteriorly related channels on the superficial part of the body. The superficial collaterals are the collaterals distributed over and emerging in the superficial areas of the body. And, the minute collaterals are the finest collaterals, which are said to have the functions of storing strange pathogens and are where the defensive Qi and the nutritive Qi flow in *Qi Xue Lun* (Treatise on Acupoints) in *Su Wen* (The Plain Questions).

Both the muscular regions and the cutaneous regions are the tendons, muscles and skins attached to the twelve regular channels. According to the meridian theory, the muscular regions are the system composed of muscles, tendons and joints where Qi of the twelve regular channels meets and connects and is distributed. They are attached to the twelve regular channels and thus are known as the twelve muscular regions. The muscular regions function to link up

110

limbs and bones and govern the movements of joints. Skin of the whole body is where the functional activities of the twelve regular channels are reflected and where Qi of the twelve regular channels goes, so it is divided into twelve parts to be connected with the twelve regular channels, and thus they are called the twelve cutaneous regions.

The Twelve Regular Channels

1. The nomenclature of the twelve regular channels

Distributed on the bilateral sides of the human body symmetrically, the twelve regular channels travel in the medial or lateral aspect of the upper or lower limbs, each of the twelve regular channels connecting with and pertaining to a Zang and a Fu organ respectively. Therefore, each of them is named after the hand or foot, Yin or Yang and Zang or Fu organ. The hand channels run to the upper limbs and the foot channel to the lower limbs; the Yin channels to the medial aspects of the limbs and pertaining to Zang organs, and the Yang channels to the lateral aspects of the limbs and pertaining to the Fu organs. See the following table for nomenclature of the twelve regular channels.

| | Yin Meridian | Yang Meridian | Distribution | |
			Yin Medial Side	Yang Lateral Side
Hand	Lung	Large Intestine	upper limbs	anterior border
	Pericardium	Triple Jiao		middle border
	Heart	Small Intestine		posterior border
Foot	Spleen	Stomach	Lower limbs	anterior border
	Liver	Gallbladder		middle border
	Kidney	Bladder		posterior border

111

2. Laws of trends, connexion and distribution, the interior-exterior relationship and the cyclical flow of Qi

(1) The trends and connexion law of the twelve regular channels: Some laws can be found concerning the trends and connexion of the twelve regular channels. According to descriptions in *Ni Shun Fei Shou* (Flow of Qi and Blood and Body Physiques) of *Ling Shu* (The Miraculous Pivot), the three Yin channels of hands go from the chest to the tips of the fingers where they connect with the three Yang channels of hands; the three Yang channels of hands run from the tips of the fingers to the head or face, where they connect with the three Yang channels of feet; the three Yang channels of feet go from the face or head to the tips of toes where they meet with the three Yin channels of feet; and the three Yin channels of feet go from the tips of toes to the abdomen or the chest where they connect with the three Yin channels of hands. So, the Yin and Yang channels connect each other to form the cycle for flow of Qi and Blood.

As the three Yang channels of hands end at the head and the three Yang channels of feet start from the head, they connect with each other on the head or face, so the head or face is said to be where all Yang channels meet.

(2) Distribution law: Distribution of the twelve regular channels on the surface of the body also have some laws to follow. In the limbs, the three Yin channels run in the medial aspect, while the three Yang channels in the lateral aspect. Generally speaking, Taiyin and Yangming channels go on the anterior border, Jueyin and Shaoyang go on the midline and Shaoyin and Taiyang go along the posterior border. In the head, Yangming channel runs on the face or forehead, Taiyang channel goes along the cheeks, vertex and the back, and Shaoyang channel runs on the bilateral sides. In the trunk, the three Yang channels of hands pass through the scapular region, the foot Yangming channel goes over the front (the chest and the abdomen), the foot Taiyang channel runs over the back and the Shaoyang channel over the bilateral sides. All the three Yin channels go through the axillary fossa, and all the three Yin channels of feet run over the abdomen. Of the channels distributed over

the abdomen, the foot Shaoyin channels goes along the first line lateral to the midline, the foot Yangming channels along the second line, the foot Taiyin along the third line and the foot Jueyin along the fourth line.

(3) The interior-exterior relationship: The three Yin channels and the three Yang channels of hands or feet, through the communication of their branches and major collaterals, form six pairs of interior-exterior relationships. That is, the foot Taiyang channel is interior-exteriorly related to the foot Shaoyin channel, the foot Shaoyang channel to the Foot Jueyin channel, the foot Yangming channel to the foot Taiyin channel, the hand Taiyang channel to the hand Shaoyin channel, the hand Shoyang channel to the hand Jueyin channel, and the hand Yangming channel to the hand Taiyin channel.

The interior-exteriorly related channels communicate in the ends of the four limbs, and travel on the corresponding positions on the medial aspect and the lateral aspect of the four limbs respectively. The Liver Channel of Foot-Jueyin, however, goes along the anterior border in the medial aspect of the legs below the point eight *cun* above the medial malleolus while the Spleen Channel of Foot-Taiyin along the midline. Above the point, the Spleen Channel goes on the anterior line while the Liver Channel goes on the midline. The interior-exteriorly related channels connect with and pertain to the Zang or Fu organs with the interior-exterior relationship respectively. For example, the Bladder Channel of Foot-Taiyang pertains to the Bladder and connects with the Kidney, the Kidney Channel of Foot-Shaoyin pertains to the Kidney and connects with the Bladder, etc.

With the direct connection of the two channels interior-exteriorly related , the relations between them are strengthened. Besides, as these two channels pertain to and connect with the same pair of Zang and Fu organs, the Zang and Fu organs with the interior-exterior relationships must be well coordinated physiologically and influence by each other pathologically. For example, the Spleen and the Stomach must well cooperate to perform the digestion and absorption of foodstuff, the Heart Fire may go to the Small Intestine, etc.

In treatment of disease, acupoints of the interior-exteriorly related channels may be adopted interchangeably. For example, acupoints of the Lung channel can be used to treat disease of the Large Intestine or its channel.

(4) Cyclical flow of Qi in the twelve regular channels: The twelve regular channels are distributed in both the interior and the exterior of the human body. Qi and Blood in the channels flow cyclically from one channel to another in sequence. They start to flow from the Lung Channel of Hand-Taiyin, passing through the channels in order, they reach the Liver Channels of Foot-Jueyin, where they enter the Lung Channel of Hand-Taiyin again to resume the second cycle. The cyclical flow of Qi and Blood in the twelve regular channels are as follows:

→the Lung Channel→the Large Intestine Channel
the Spleen Channel←the Stomach Channel←
→the Heart Channel→the Small Intestine Channel
the Kidney Channel←the Bladder Channel←
→Pericardium Channel→the Triple Jiao Channel
the Liver Channel←the Gallbladder Channel←

3. Distribution of the twelve regular channels

(1) The Lung Channel of Hand-Taiyin: The Lung Channel of Hand-Taiyin originates from the Middle Jiao, running downward to connect with the Large Intestine. Winding back, it goes along the lower orifice (the duodenum) and the upper orifice (the cardia) of the Stomach, passes through the diaphragm, and enters the Lung, its pertaining organ. Then it goes upward to the throat where it runs transversely to the laterosuperior side of the chest. Emerging in the axillary fossa, it runs downward along the anterior border of the medial aspect of the upper arm, passes through the cubital fossa and enters Cunkou (the radial artery at the wrist for pulse palpation). Passing through the thenar eminence, it reaches the tip of the thumb (Shaoshang, LU 11)..

The branch proximal to the wrist emerges from Lieque (LU 7) and runs directly to the radial side of the tip of the index finger (Shangyang, LI 1) where it links with the Large Intestine Channel of Hand-Yangming.

(2) The Large Intestine Channel of Hand-Yangming: The Large Intestine Channel starts from the tip of the radial side of the index finger (Shangyang, LI 1). Passing through the dorsum of hand, it travels along the anterior border of the lateral aspect of the arm to the shoulder. Then it goes in front of the shoulder joint backward to the point below the spinous process of the 7th cervical vertebra (Dazhui, DU 14). From there, it goes forwards, entering the supraclavicular fossa to connect with the Lung in the thorax. Descending, it passes through the diaphragm to reach the Large Intestine, its pertaining organ.

The branch emerging in the supraclavicular fossa goes upward along the side of the neck and the cheek to enter the lower gum. Winding back, it runs around the corners of mouth and crosses the opposite channel at philtrum, ending at the opposite side of the nose (Yingxiang, LI 20), where it links with the Stomach Channel of Hand-Yangming.

(3) The Stomach Channel of Foot-Yangming: The Stomach Channel of Foot-Yangming starts from the lateral side of ala nasi (Yingxiang, LI 20). It then ascends along the side of the nose to the bridge of the nose where it goes laterally to enter the inner canthus to meet with the Bladder Channel of Foot-Taiyang. Turning downwards along the lateral side of the nose, it enters the upper gum. Reemerging, it curves around the lips and descends to meet the opposite channel at the mentaolabial groove (Chengjiang, RN 24). Then it goes posterolaterally across the portion of the cheek at Daying (ST 5). Winding back along the mandible, it ascends in front of the ear and transverses Shangguan (GL 3). Then it follows the anterior hairline and reaches the forehead.

The facial branch emerging in front of Daying (ST 5) runs downwards to Renying (ST 9). From there, it goes along the throat posteriorly to Dazhui (DU 14). Then it Winds back and enters the supraclavicular fossa. Descending, it passes through the diaphragm, enters the Stomach, its pertaining organ and connects with the Spleen.

The straight portion of the channel arises from the supraclavicular fossa. It runs downwards, passing through the nipple. It then descends by the umbilicus and enters Qichong (ST 30) on the groin.

The branch from the lower orifice of the Stomach descends inside the abdomen and joints the previous portion of the channel at Qichong (ST 30). Then it runs downwards along the anterior aspect of the thin, reaching the knee. Descending further, it goes along the anterior border of the lateral aspect of the tibia, passes through the dorsum of foot and enters the lateral side of the tip of the second toe.

The tibial branch arises from Zusanli (ST 36), three *cun* below the knee, and enters the lateral side of the third toe.

The branch from the dorsum of the foot emerges from Chongyang (ST 42), ending at the medial side of the tip of the greater toe (Yinbai SP 1), where it links with the Spleen Channel of Foot-Taiyin.

(4) The Spleen Channel of Foot-Taiyin: The Spleen Channel of Foot-Taiyin starts from the medial side of the greater toe (Yinbai SP 1). It runs along the medial aspect of the foot at the junction of the red and white skin, and ascends in front of the medial malleolus up to the leg, where it goes along the midline of the medial aspect of the leg. At the point eight *cun* above the medial malleolus, it crosses and goes in front of the Liver Channel of the Foot-Jueyin . Passing through the anterior medial aspect of the thigh, it enters the abdomen, then the Spleen, its pertaining organ and connects with the Stomach. From there it ascends, passing through the diaphragm and running alongside the esophagus. When it reaches the root of the tongue, it spreads over its lower surface.

The branch from the Stomach goes upward through the diaphragm, and flows into the Heart to link with the Heart Channel of Hand-Shaoyin.

(5) The Heart Channel of Hand-Shaoyin: The Heart Channel of Hand-Shaoyin starts from the Heart. Emerging, it spreads over the "Heart system". Passing through the diaphragm, it goes downward to connect with the Small Intestine.

The branch emerging from the Heart system goes alongside the

116

esophagus upwards to connect with the "eye system".

The straight portion of the channel arises from the Heart system, then it goes upwards to the Lung, where it turns downwards and e-merges from the axilla (Jiquan, HT 1). Going along the posterior border of the medial aspect of the upper arm, it passes through the tip of the elbow and reaches the pisiform region proximal to the palm. Then it follows the medial aspect of the little finger to its tip (Shaochong, HT 9) and links with the Small Intestine Channel of Hand-Taiyang.

(6) The Small Intestine Channel of Hand-Shaoyang: The Small Intestine Channel of Hand-Shaoyang originates from the ulnar side of the little finger (Shaoze, SI 1). Going along the posterior border of the dorsum of hand and the lateral aspect of the forearm, it pass-es through the elbow to the posterior border of the shoulder joint. From there, it runs around the scapula to meet the opposite channel at Dazhui (DU 14). Then it travels forwards to enter the supraclav-icular fossa. Inside the body cavities, it connects with the Heart, and alongside the esophagus, it passes through the diaphragm to the Stomach, where it continues to descend to the Small Intestine, its pertaining organ.

The branch from the supraclavicular fossa reaches the cheek along the neck, then it ascends to the outer canthus and goes backwards to enter the ear (Tinggong, SI 19).

The branch from the cheek ascends to the infraorbital region and further to the inner canthus (Jingming, BD 1), where it links with the Bladder Channel of Foot-Taiyang.

(7) The Bladder Channel of Foot-Taiyang: The Bladder Channel of Foot-Taiyang starts at the inner canthus (Jingming, BD 1). As-cending to the forehead, it joins its opposite channel at the vertex (Baihui, DU 20).

The branch arising from the vertex goes to the temple.

The straight portion of the channel goes backward and downward to the occipital region to enter and communicate with the brain. Turning back, it descends to the posterior aspect of the neck, meet-ing its opposite channel at Dazhui (DU 14). Then it bifurcates and

117

travels 1. 5 *cun* lateral to the medial side of the scapula and the spinal column, reaching the lumbar region, where it enters the body cavity via the paravertebral muscle to connect with the Kidney and join the Bladder, its pertaining organ.

The branch arising from the lumbar region descends beside the spinal column. Passing through the gluteal region, it travels downwards to the popliteal fossa along the lateral side of the posterior aspect of the thigh.

The branch originating from the posterior aspect of the neck goes in the medial side of the scapular region. At Fufen (UB 41), it runs downwards 3 *cun* lateral to the spinal column to the hip joint. Then it goes along the posterior aspect of the thigh to meet the previous branch in the popliteal fossa. Going further downwards, it passes through the gastrocnemius muscle and emerges behind the external malleolus. From there, it runs along the lateral border of the dorsum of foot to terminates at the tip of the lateral side of the little toe (Zhiyin, KD 1), where it links with the Kidney Channel of Foot-Shaoyin.

(8) The Kidney Channel of Foot-Shaoyin: The Kidney Channel of Foot-Shaoyin starts from the inferior aspect of the small toe and runs obliquely to the sole (Yongquan, KI 1). Emerging from the lower aspect of the tubersity of the navicular bone, it runs behind the medial malleolus and enters the heel. Then it ascends along posterior border of the medial side of the leg to the medial side of the popliteal fossa and further upward along the postero-medial aspect of the thigh towards the spinal column (Changqiang, DU 1). Passing through the spinal column, it enters the Kidney, its pertaining organ, and connects with the Bladder.

The straight portion of the channel goes upwards from the Kidney. Passing through the Liver and the diaphragm, it enters the Lung and alongside the throat, reaches the bilateral sides of the root of the tongue.

The branch arising from the Lung connects with the Heart and flows into the thorax to link with the Pericardium Channel of Hand-Jueyin.

118

(9) The Pericardium Channel of Hand-Jueyin: The Pericardium Channel of Hand-Jueyin originates from the thorax. Emerging, it communicates with the pericardium, its pertaining organ. Passing through the diaphragm, it connects with the Upper Jiao, the Middle Jiao and the Lower Jiao successively.

The branch arising from the thorax emerges from the costal region 3 *cun* below anterior axillary fossa (Tianchi, PC 1). It then ascends to the axilla and travels along the midline of the medial aspect of the upper arm to enter the cubital fossa. Passing through the wrist, it enters the center of the palm (Laogong, PC 8) and further goes along the radial side of the middle finger to its tip (Zhongchong, PC 9).

The branch from the palm goes to the tip of the ring finger along its ulnar side to link with the Triple Jiao Channel of Hand-Shaoyang.

(10) The Triple Jiao Channel of Hand-Shaoyang: The Triple Jiao Channel of Hand-Shaoyang starts from the ulnar side of the tip of the ring finger (Guanchong, SJ 1). Going upwards along the ulnar side of the ring finger, it reaches the dorsum of the hand. Then it goes upward between the ulna and the radius in the forearm. Passing through the olecranon and along the lateral aspect of the upper arm, it enters the supraclavicular fossa from the shoulder, spreads over the thorax to connect with the pericardium. Passing through the diaphragm, it communicates with the Upper Jiao, the Middle Jiao and the Lower Jiao successively.

The branch from the thorax goes upwards to emerge in the supraclavicular fossa. Reaching the shoulder, it meets its opposite channel at Dazhui (DU 14). Then, it ascends to the posterior aspect of the neck where along the posterior region of the ear, it goes up to the temple. Then it curves downwards. Passing through the cheek, it reaches the inferorbital region.

The branch arising from the posterior region of the ear enters the ear and reemerges in front of the ear. Crossing the previous branch in cheek, it terminates at the outer canthus (Tongziliao, GB 1) to link with the Gallbladder Channel of Foot-Shaoyang.

119

(11) The Gallbladder Channel of Foot-Shaoyang: The Gallbladderr Channel of Foot-Shaoyang originates from the outer canthus (Tongziliao, GB 1), ascends to the corner of the forehead (Hanyan, GB 4), then curves downwards to the retroauricular region (Wangu, GB 12). From there, it ascends and curves, passing through the forehead, to the supraorbital region, curves backward and downward to the retroauricular region again (Fengchi, GB 20) and runs along the side of the neck to the shoulder. Then it meets its opposite at Dazhui (DU 14) and runs forward to enter the supraclavicular fossa.

The branch from the retroauricular region enters the ear and reemerges in front of the ear, reaching the posterior border of the outer canthus.

The branch arising from the outer canthus runs downwards and meets the branch of the Triple Jiao Channel of Hand-Shaoyang at Daying (GB ST 5), then it goes to the infraorbital region. The branch going downward passes through the mandible of the jaw and the neck, meeting the previous channel in the supraclavicular fossa. Then, it enters the body cavity. Passing through the diaphragm, it connects with the Liver and reaches the Gallbladder, its pertaining organ. From there, it runs inside the hypochondriac region. Coming out from the groin, it runs along the margin of the pubic hair and transverses to the hip region (Huantiao, GB 30).

The straight portion of the channel runs downward from the supraclavicular fossa, passes in front of the axilla along the lateral aspect of the chest and through the free end of the ribs to the hip region where it meets the previous branch. Then it descends along the lateral aspect of the thigh to the lateral side of the knee. Going further downward along the anterior border of the fibula all the way to its lower end, it emerges from the anterior aspect of the external malleolus and follows the dorsum of the foot to the lateral side of the tip of the 4th toe (Zuqiaoyin, GB 44).

The branch from the dorsum (Zulingqi, GB 41) of the foot goes forwards to the lateral aspect of the big toe, then it turns back, passing through the nail, and terminates at its hairy region, where it links with the Liver Channel of Foot-Jueyin.

(12) The Liver Channel of Foot-Jueyin: The Liver Channel of Foot-Jueyin originates from the hairy region of the great toe. Running upward along the dorsum of the foot, passing through Zhongfeng (LR 4), which is 1 *cun* in front of the medial malleolus, it ascends to an area 8 *cun* above the medial malleolus, where it runs across and behind the Spleen Channel of Foot-Taiyin. Then it runs further upwards to the medial aspect of the knee and along the medial aspect of the thigh to enter the pubic hairy region, where it curves around the external genital and goes up to the lower abdomen. It then runs upward alongside the Stomach to reach the Liver, its pertaining organ and connects with the Gallbladder. From there, it continues to ascend, passing through the diaphragm and branching out from the costal and hypochondriac region. Then it runs upwards along the posterior aspect of the throat, entering the nasopharharynx and connects with the "eye system". Running upwards further, it emerges from the forehead and , goes upward further and meets the Du Channel at the vertex.

The branch from the eye system runs downward into the cheek, and curves around the inner surface of the lips.

The branch arising from the Liver, passing through the diaphragm, goes upward to enter the Lung, linking with the Lung Channel of Hand-Taiyin.

The Eight
Extraordinary Channels

The eight extraordinary channels are a collective term for the Du Channel, the Ren Channel, the Chong Channel, the Dai Channel, the Yinwei Channel, the Yangwei Channel, the Yinqiao Channel and the Yangqiao Channel. Different from the twelve regular channels, they are not so regular in distribution, have neither direct connecting or pertaining relations with the Zang Fu organs nor interior-exterior relationships among them, hence they are so called.

The eight extraordinary channels, traveling vertically and transversely among the twelve regular channels, have three functions: ① Strengthening the relations among the twelve regular channels. For example, the Du Channel can govern all the Yang channels; the Ren Channel controls all the Yin channels; the Chong Channel which is distributed up to the head and down to the feet, can receive Qi and Blood of all the three Yin channels and the three Yang channels; and the Dai Channel has the effect of controlling all the channels running vertically by communicating with the channels passing through the abdomen and the lumbar region, the Yinwei Channel maintains and links with the three Yang channels of both hands and feet, and the Yinwei Channel maintains and links with the Yin channels of hand and foot. ② Regulating Qi and Blood in the twelve regular channels. When Qi and Blood in the twelve regular channels are abundant, they may partly flow to the eight extraordinary channels to be stored; while when Qi and Blood in the twelve regular channels are insufficient, Qi and Blood will flow from the eight extraordinary channels to the twelve regular channels. ③ Being closely related to the Liver, the Kidney, the uterus, the brain and the marrow. In other words, the eight extraordinary channels have some relationships in physiology and pathology with the above mentioned organs.

1. The Du Channel

(1) Distribution: The Du Channel originates from the uterus and goes downward. Emerging from the perineum, it runs posteriorly along the interior of the spinal column to Fengfu (DU 16), where it enters the intracranial cavity to connect with the brain. It further ascends to the vertex along the posterior midline of the head from the nape. Passing through the forehead, the nose and the upper lips, it terminates at the frenulum of the superior lip.

The branch from the spinal column enters the abdominal cavity to connect with the Kidney.

The branch arising from the lower abdomen ascends straightly inside the abdomen. Passing through the umbilicus and the Heart, it runs to the throat and further to the jaw, where it goes around the lips, reaching the midpoints of the infraorbital regions of the eyes.

(2) Functions:

① Being the sea of the Yang channels: The Du Channel runs along the midline of the back, a Yang region of the body, and meets with the three Yang channels of both hand and foot and the Yangwei Channel repeatedly, so it can govern all the Yang channels of the body and hence the saying.

② Being closely related to the brain, spinal column and the Kidney: The Du Channel runs inside the spinal column and connects with the brain, so it has a close relationship with the brain and the spinal column. In addition, the Du Channel originates from the uterus and pertains to the Kidney, so it also has a close relationship with the Kidney and the reproductive ability of the human body, especially the reproductive ability of male. Doctors throughout history mostly adopted the methods of tonifying the Du Channel to treat disturbance of the reproductive function.

2. The Ren Channel

(1) Distribution: The Ren Channel originates from the uterus. Emerging from the perineum, it goes anteriorly to the pubic region. Then it runs upwards along the anterior midline of the body to the throat, where it ascends further to the jaw, runs around the lips to the infraorbital regions along the cheek.

(2) Functions:

① Being the sea of the Yin channels: The Ren Channel runs along the midline of the anterior of the body, which is a Yin area, and meets frequently with the three Yin channels of both hand and foot and the Yinwei channels, so it can control all the Yin channels of the body and hence the saying.

② Dominating pregnancy: The Ren Channel originates from the uterus and controls all the Yin channels. As the fetus can be well nourished only when Qi and Blood in the Ren Channels flow smoothly and Qi and Blood in the Chong Channel is fully filled, so it is said that the Ren Channel controls pregnancy.

3. The Chong Channel

(1) Distribution: The Chong Channel starts from the uterus. E-merging from the perineum, it runs together with the Kidney Channel of Foot-Shaoyin at the groin. Then it ascends alongside the umbilicus and spreads over the chest. Going further upward, it passes through the throat, runs around the lips and terminates in the infraorbital regions.

The branch originates from the Kidney together with the Major Collaterals of the Foot-Shaoyin. Running downward, it emerges at the inguinal region and then enters the popliteal fossa along the medial aspect of the thigh. From there, it descends further along the interior border of the tibia to the posterior aspect of the medial malleolus, entering the sole. The branch from the posterior aspect of the medial malleolus goes anteriorly ad obliquely to the dorsum of foot, reaching the great toe.

The branch arising from the uterus goes backward to communicate with the Du Channel, and then runs inside the spinal column.

(2) Functions:

① Regulating Qi and Blood in the twelve regular channels: The Chong Channel runs upwards to the head and downward to the sole, so it communicates with all the body, and functions to regulate Qi and Blood in the twelve regular channel. This is why it is called the sea of the twelve regular channels.

② Being closely related to the female reproductive ability: Originating from the uterus, the Chong Channel is where Qi and Blood are fully filled. Thus, only when Qi and Blood are sufficient in the Chong Channel and flow smoothly in the Ren Channel can a female has a regular menstruation and a normal reproductive ability.

4. The Dai Channel

(1) Distribution: The Dai Channel originates from the hypochondriac region, then it runs downward and forward to the Damai point (GB 26) and goes around the waist. The portion of the channel in the front droops to the lower abdomen.

(2) Functions:

Going around the waist like a belt, the Dai Channel mainly functions to tighten the channels distributing vertically. Besides, it is also suggested that the Dai Channel has the function of consolidating pregnancy.

5. The Yinqiao Channel and the Yangqiao Channel

(1) Distributions: This kind of channels exist on the left and right of the body respectively, both originating below the malleolus.

The Yinqiao Channel originates from Zhaohai (KD 6). It ascends along the posterior aspect of the medial malleolus to the medial aspect of the lower limb. Passing through the external genital, abdomen and chest, it enters the supraclavicular fossa. Then it emerges in front of Renying (ST 9), going upward alongside the nose to reach the inner canthus where it meets with the Taiyang channels of both hand and foot and the Yangqiao Channel.

The Yangqiao Channel starts from Shenmai (BD 62) below the medial malleolus. Then it ascends in the posterior aspect of the external malleolus. Passing through posterolateral aspects of the abdomen and the chest and the lateral aspect of the should and neck, it goes around the corner of the mouth and reaches the inner canthus, where it links with the Taiyang channels of both hand and foot and the Yinqiao Channel. From there, it continues to ascend, enters the hair and then curves downwards to the retroauricular region and meets the Gallbladder Channel of Foot-Shaoyang on the nape.

(2) Functions: The Yinqiao Channel and the Yangqiao Channel function collectively to control the movement of the lower limbs to keep the movement to be quick. Besides, they also have the function of nourishing the eyes and controlling the opening-closing movement of the eyes. In the ancient times, they are also said to have the function of controlling the left and right of the human body respectively.

6. The Yinwei Channel and the Yangwei Channel

(1) Distribution: The Yinwei Channel starts from the point where the three Yin channels of foot meet in the medial aspect of the leg. It then ascends along the medial aspect of the lower limb to the abdomen, where it runs together with the Spleen Channel of Foot-Taiyin to the costal region. From the costal region, it ascends together with the Liver Channel of Foot-Jueyin to the throat to meet

125

the Ren Channel.

The Yangwei Channel originates below the external malleolus. Then it goes upwards with the Gallbladder Channel of Foot-Shaoyang. Passing through the lateral aspect of the lower limbs and the posterolateral aspect of the trunk, it ascends to the shoulder from the posterior aspect of the axilla. From there, it runs upward along the neck and the retroauricular region to the forehead, spreading over the side of head and the posterior aspect of the neck, meeting the Du Channel.

(2) Functions: The Yinwei Channel functions to maintain and connect all the Yin channels of the body, while the Yangwei Channel, to maintain and connect all the Yang channels of the body.

Branches of the Twelve Regular Channels, Major Collaterals, Muscular Regions and Cutaneous Regions

1. The branches of the twelve regular channels

Branches of channels refer to the regular channels separating from the twelve regular channels. They are the important branches of the twelve regular channels distributing over the chest, abdomen, lumbar region and the head.

(1) Features of distribution: All the branches of the channels derive from the pertaining channels above the knees and elbows at the four limbs, known as "separating". Then they enter the depth of the Zang Fu organs, known as "entering". Emerging, they go upward to the head and face, which is known as "emerging". While the branches of the Yin channels ascend to the head and face, they enter the six Yang channels, known as "combining". Therefore, features of the branches of the channels can be summarized as "separating", "entering", "emerging" and "combining". There are six pairs of branches which are composed of the branches of the interi-

or-exterioly related channels. That is, the branches of the Foot-Taiyang and the branch of the Foot-Shaoyin form one pair, the branches of the Foot-Shaoyang and that of the Foot-Jueyin form one pair, that of the Foot-Yangming and that of the Foot-Taiyin form one pair, that of the Hand-Taiyang and that of the Hand-Shaoyin form one pair, that of the Hand-Shaoyang and that of the Hand-Yueyin form one pair, and that of the Hand-Yangming and that of Hand-Taiyin form one pair. Their concrete distribution is omitted here.

(2) Physiological functions:

① Strengthening the connections of the interior-exteriorly related channels within the body: Entering the body cavities, the branches of the interior-exteriorly related channels run parallelly, pass through the interior-exteriorly related Zang Fu organs, and when e-merging, branches of the Yin channels combine with the branches of the Yang channels to flow together to the Yang channels on the ex-terior. Thus, they have the function of strengthening the connec-tions of the interior-exteriorly related channels in the body cavities.

② Strengthening the central connection between the exterior and the interior of the human body and that between the four limbs and the trunk: As all the branches of channels originate from their per-taining channels at the knees or elbows of the limbs and go towards the Heart when they enter the body cavity, informations can be transmitted from the exterior to the interior of the human body, and thus the connecting effect of the channels is extended.

③ Strengthening the connection of the twelve regular channels with the head: Of the twelve regular channels, it is mainly the six Yang channels that reach the head, however, all the branches of the twelve regular channels arrive at head. So they have the function of strengthening the connections of the twelve regular channels with the head.

④ Extending the areas the twelve regular channels connect: Some of the branches of the twelve regular channels runs to where their pertaining channels don't. So, the areas connecting with the chan-nels are extended and correspondingly, indications of the channels are also extended.

⑤ Strengthening the connections of the three Yin channels and the three Yang channels of foot with the Heart: The branches of the three Yin channels and the three Yang channels of foot ascend through the abdomen and the chest to connect with the Heart, so they can be used to analyze the relations between the Zang Fu organs in the abdominal cavity and the Heart in both physiology and pathology.

2. The major collaterals

The major collaterals also branch off from the twelve regular channels and are mainly distributed over the surface of the body. There are fifteen major collaterals in number, the major collaterals of the twelve regular channels, that of the Du and Ren Channels and that of the Spleen. Sometimes the major collaterals of the Stomach is also included and so it is also called the sixteen major collaterals.

The major collaterals are the major part of the collateral system. They function to lead all the minute or fine collaterals of the whole body. The fine collaterals deriving from the major collaterals are named minute collaterals, while the collaterals distributed over the surface, the superficial collaterals.

(1) Feature of distribution: The fifteen major collaterals have their own characteristics in distribution. That is, the major collaterals of the twelve regular channels all start below the knees or elbows at the four limbs, and the major collaterals of the interior-exteriorly related channels connect with each other, the major collaterals of the Yin channels go to these of their related channels and vice versa. The major collaterals of the Ren Channel is distributed over the abdomen, that of the Du Channel over the back, and that of the Spleen over the side of the body.

(2) Functions:

① Strengthening connections between the interior-exteriorly related channels: This is mainly realized by the major collaterals of the Yin channels running to the Yang channels and these of the Yang channels to the Yin channels, so the connections of the interior-exteriorly related channels are strengthened on the four limbs. Although some major collaterals go to the Zang Fu organs to connect with them, they haven't direct pertaining-connecting relations with the Zang Fu organs.

② Leading all the other collaterals of the body and strengthening the connections of the front, the back and the side of the body: All the other collaterals including the minute collaterals and the superficial collaterals derive from the major collaterals, so the major collaterals have a leading effect on them. Besides, as the major collateral is mainly distributed over the abdominal aspect of the body, that of the Du Channel over the back of the body and that of the Spleen over the side of the body, the major collaterals also have the function of unifying the front, the back and the side of the human body.

③ Transpoting Qi and Blood to nourish the whole body: The collaterals branch off gradually, distributed over the whole body like a net to touch the peripheral tissues, so Qi and Blood in the channels can pass through the major collaterals, the minute collaterals and the superficial collaterals to all the tissues to perform their nourishing effect.

3. The muscular regions

Muscular regions refer to the tendons and muscles attached to the twelve regular channels. They depend on the nourishment of the Qi and Blood in the twelve regular channels for their movements and are regulated by the twelve regular channels, so they are classified as twelve parts, known as the twelve muscular regions.

(1) Features of distribution: Distribution of the muscular regions are about the same with the distribution of the twelve regular channels on the surface. Generally speaking, the muscular regions mostly run on the superficial parts, from the limbs to the head or the trunk, and usually accumulate around the joints or bones. Some of then enters the thoracic and the abdominal cavities, but they don't connect with Zang Fu organs. The muscular regions of the three Yang channels of both hand and foot are mainly distributed over the lateral aspects of the limbs, while these of the three Yin channels over the medial aspects of the limbs.

(2) Functions: The main physiological functions of the muscular

regions are to link up with the four limbs and the bones, connect with bones and control the movement of joints.

4. The cutaneous regions

The cutaneous regions are the distinct cutaneous regions classified in accordance with the twelve regular channels. The twelve regular channels and their collaterals run in certain areas on the surface of the body, consequently, all the skin of the body can be classified as twelve portions, known as the twelve cutaneous regions.

The cutaneous regions are both the cutaneous regions classified in accordance with the distribution of the twelve regular channels and their collaterals on the surface of the body and the twelve areas where Qi of the twelve regular channels are distributed. Therefore, pathogens may be transmitted to the channels and further to the Zang Fu organs through the cutaneous regions. On the other hand, disorders of the channels can also be reflected on the cutaneous regions. In the clinic, observation of the colour and luster of the different cutaneous regions may help to diagnose the different diseases of the channels or Zang Fu organs. Application of such therapies as ointment, moxibustion and hot compress on the cutaneous regions can treat diseases of some Zang Fu organs.

Physiology of Meridians and the Clinical Application of Meridian Theory

1. Physiological functions of the meridians

The functions of the meridian are also known as Jing Qi, which possess the following four aspects:

(1) Linking the exterior with the interior, the upper with the lower, and connecting with Zang Fu organs: Being different in physiological functions, the Five Zang organs, the Six Fu organs, the limbs, the bones, the five sensory organs, the nine orifices, the

skin, the muscles, the tendons and the bones of the human body carry out the organic wholistic activities in harmony, ensuring that the upper, the lower, the interior and the exterior of the human body to be unified and harmonized and that the human body to be an organic unity. This kind of organic connection and coordination mainly depend on the connecting and communicating effects of the meridians. The twelve regular channels and their branches travel transversely and vertically, reaching the exterior as well as the interior, the upper as well as the lower of the human body and connecting with or pertaining to Zang Fu organs. The eight extraordinary channels connect and communicate with the twelve regular channels, and the twelve muscular regions and the twelve cutaneous regions link with the tendons, vessels, skin and musles. So the Zang Fu organs and the tissues of the human body are closely connected with each other, and the human body is organized to be an organic whole in which its different parts are kept in harmony in the functional activities of the whole body. The connecting effect of the meridians are mainly manifested as four aspects: ① linking the Zang Fu organs with the limbs; ②linking the Zang Fu organs with the sensory organs and the orifices; ③ connecting one organ with others; and ④ connecting one meridian with other meridians.

(2) Transporting Qi and Blood to nourish the whole body: All the Zang Fu organs and tissues of the human body depend on the nourishment of Qi and Blood for their normal physiological functions, and it is the meridians that send Qi and Blood to the Zang Fu organs and tissues to nourish them, fight against pathogens and protect the human body. Just as stated in *Ben Zang* (On Organs) of *Ling Shu* (The Miraculous Pivot): "Meridians are where Qi and Blood flow and thus they have the function of regulating Yin and Yang, moistening tendons and bones and promoting movement of joints."

(3) Transmitting and conducting effect: This means that the meridians can response to such stimuli as needling and transmit the sense caused by the needling. The gaining of Qi and a sense of flow of Qi in acupuncture, for example, are just the manifestations of the

transmitting and conducting effect of the meridians.

(4) Regulating balance of the human body: The meridians can keep the functional activities of the human body in balance because they carry Qi and Blood to balance Yin and Yang. When Qi and Blood are not in harmony or Yin and Yang are not balanced due to diseases, acupuncture or moxibustion can be employed to stimulate the meridians to perform their regulating effect. Experiments proved that needling on some acupoints may exert a favorable double-way regulatory effects on the functional activities. In other words, it can inhibit the hyperactivity and excite the hypofunctions.

2. Application of the meridians theory

(1) Explaining pathological changes: Physiologically, the meridians have the effect of carrying Qi and Blood and conducting and transmitting sense caused by stimuli. In pathology, they may be where the pathogens are transmitted and where the pathological changes are reflected. This includes: ① pathogens attacking the exterior may go deeper or even to the Zang Fu organs through the meridians; ② diseases of the internal organs may be reflected on the surface of the body through the transmitting effect of the meridians; and ③ diseases may be transmitted among Zang Fu organs.

(2) Guiding diagnosis and treatment of diseases:

① Guiding diagnosis of disease: As the meridians travel to certain regions and connect with or pertain to certain Zang Fu organs, doctors may determine the location and nature of a disease in accordance with both the location of the symptoms or signs of the disease and the distribution of the meridians as well as the Zang Fu organs that the meridians connect with. For instance, headache marked by pain in the forehead is mostly related to Yangming channel; pain on the temporal region is usually related to Shanyang channel; pain on the back of head and the vertex is mostly indicative of disorders of the Taiyang channel; and pain in the vertex is mostly related to diseases of the Jueyin channels; and pain in the bilateral costal regions mostly indicates disease of the Liver or the Gallbladder. It is found in the clinic that tenderness, nodular or streak masses and morphological changes are often exhibited in the places where the meridians travel or the acupoints which collect Qi of meridians, which can help to diagnose diseases. For example, Lung disease often presents nodular mass in Feishu (BD 13) or ternderness in Zhongfu (LU 1).

② Guiding treatment: The meridians theory is widely applied in the clinical treatment of diseases, and is of great guiding significance for such therapies as acupuncture and moxibustion therapy, massage therapy and drug therapy.

Acupuncture, moxibustion and massage therapy carry out the treatment by needling or massaging the points adjacent to the disease location or far away from the location on the meridians passing by the disease location, in order to regulate the functional activities of Qi and Blood in the meridians. Therefore, meridians theory is the main theoretical basis of these therapies.

Drugs can play the therapeutic effect depending on the transmitting effect of the meridians which send the drugs to where diseases occur. The ancient doctors, based on their long clinical practice, suggested the theory of "Attribution of drugs to a channel" and " Guiding drug for a channel", which have been effectively guiding the application of the drugs in accordance with their affinity to a channel or the application of the guiding drugs. For example, Qiang Huo (Rhizoma seu Radix Notopterygii)) should be used in the case of headache ascribed to Taiyang channel, Bai Zhi (Radix Angelicae Dahuricae) in the case of headache ascribed to the Yangming channel, and Chai Hu (Radix Bupleuri) in the case of headache ascribed to Shaoyang channel.

Such therapies that are widely used in the clinic today as acupuncture anaesthesia, auricular needling, electro-acupuncture, etc. , are all developed on the basis of the meridian theory.

Etiology and Mechanism of Occurrence of Disease

T CM believes that man is an organic unity with the Five Zang organs as its core realized by the connecting effect of the meridians. There exist the dynamic balance maintained by the contradictive movements among the Zang Fu organs and between man and nature so that the human body can conduct its normal physiological functions. When this dynamic balance is disturbed due to various kinds of factors and the human body fails to adjust this disturbance to be normal, disease will occur as a result.

The etiological factors refer to the factors that cause disease by destroying the relative balance of the human body, which include abnormal climatic changes, infection of infectious pathogen, emotional stimuli, improper eating, over tiredness or resting, taking heavy loading, traumatic injury and insect bites. In the process of disease, the cause and the result act on each other. A result in a certain stage of disease may become the cause in another stage. For example, Phlegm and congealed Blood, on the one hand, are the pathological products generated by disturbance of the functions of

Zang Fu organs, on the other hand, are the pathological factors when they affect the functional activities of Zang Fu organs or the flow of Qi and Blood.

Pathogenic Factors

Pathogenic factor is a general term for all the factors that can disturb the balance between Yin and Yang of the human body and cause disease. Etiological theory, therefore, deals with the properties of the pathogenic factors, their influence on the structure and the functions of the human body and their features in causing diseases.

The etiological theory in TCM originated long time ago and has experienced a long period of development. In general, the pathogenic factors can be classified as three groups in accordance with their different origins, different ways of invading the body and their different features in causing disease: ① The exogenous pathogens, including the six climatic conditions in excess and the epidemic exogenous pathogens; ② the endogenous pathogens, and ③ the other pathogens including the improper eating, over working or resting, intemperance of sexual activities , traumatic injury and animal injury. This classification based on both the pathogenic factors and the ways of occurrence of disease can guide the Syndrome identification in the clinic practice.

Apart from the objective conditions that may become the pathogenic factors, TCM recognize causes of a disease mainly based on the clinical manifestations of the disease through analyzing the symptoms and signs in order to lay the basis for application of drugs, which is known as "seeking the cause of disease by analyzing the manifestations". Therefore, TCM places its emphasis on both the different natures and features of different pathogenic factors and the clinical manifestations of diseases caused by the pathogenic factors to make correct diagnosis and adopt proper treatment.

1. The six climatic conditions in excess (six exogenous pathogens)

The six climatic conditions in Excess is a general term for the pathogenic Wind, the pathogenic Cold, the pathogenic Summer Heat, the pathogenic Dampness, the pathogenic Dryness and the pathogenic Fire, the six kinds of exogenous pathogenic factors. Under normal conditions, Wind, Cold, Summer Heat, Dampness, Dryness and Fire are referred to as the six kinds of climates which are the necessary conditions for growing of everything in the world. When the weather changes abnormally or does not match with the seasons or when the weather changes suddenly while the resistant ability of the human body is lowered as a result of Deficiency of the Vital Qi, the six climatic conditions will invade the human body to cause disease, in this case, they turn to be the six kinds of exogenous pathogens.

Generally speaking, the six exogenous pathogens have the following features when they cause disease:

① Being closely related to seasons, climates and living environments: For example, disease caused by Wind is mostly seen in spring, that caused by Summer Heat is mainly seen in summer, that caused by Dampness is often detected in the long-summer and the early autumn, that caused by Dryness is mainly found in the late autumn, and that caused by Cold is mainly seen in winter. Besides, people living long in a Damp place often suffer from the disease caused by Dampness, and those working in an environments of high temperature are often affected by Dryness Heat or Fire.

② The six exogenous pathogens may attack the human body singly or in combination to cause such disease as common cold due to Wind Cold, diarrhea due to Dampness Heat and arthralgia due to Wind Cold.

③ The six exogenous pathogens, in the process of disease, not only affect each other, but also turn into each other in given conditions. For example, Cold pathogen may transform into Heat when it enters the interior of the human body, and long-standing existence of Dampness Summer Heat may transform into Dryness to impair

Yin.

④ The six exogenous pathogens are also called the six pathogens affected outside the body because they mainly go into the body through the skin or the mouth and nose or through the both.

(1) Pathogenic Wind: Wind is the prevalent climate in the spring, but it exists all the year round. So disease caused by Wind is mostly seen in the spring but they may also be seen in other seasons. Pathogenic Wind is the most important one of the six exogenous pathogens, which attacks surface of the human body first.

The nature of the pathogenic Wind and the features of disease caused by pathogenic Wind are as follows:

① Being a Yang pathogen, having an opening property and tending to attack the Yang portion of the body: Wind is mobile in nature instead of still. It turns to go upward and outward, so it is regarded as a Yang pathogen. When Wind invades the body, it often causes relaxation of the striae of muscles. As it goes upwards and outwards, it often attacks the Yang portions of the body such as the head and face, the Yang meridians and the muscles and skin, leading to opening of the striae of muscles and the ensuing headache, sweating, aversion to wind, etc. So it is said that the Yang portions of the body are most likely to be attacked by the pathogenic Wind first.

② Being mobile in nature and changing rapidly: Pathogenic Wind often causes disease marked by changeable locations. For example, the arthralgia due to pathogenic Wind is also called the migratory arthralgia because the arthralgia often migrates from one joint to another. Changing rapidly means that disease caused by Wind pathogen often has a sudden onset and variable manifestations. For example, urticaria, a disease mainly caused by pathogenic Wind, is usually manifested as itching skin and the skin lesions that occur and disappear alternately without fixed positions. In addition, diseases caused by pathogenic Wind have a sudden onset and rapid progress in most cases.

③ Being the head of the six exogenous pathogens: Pathogenic Wind is the prime pathogenic factor of all the six exogenous

137

pathogens, such pathogens as pathogenic Cold, pathogenic Dampness, pathogenic Dryness and pathogenic Fire often attach themselves to the pathogenic Wind to invade the human body, leading to diseases caused by exogenous Wind Cold, exogenous Wind Dampness or pathogenic Wind Heat. So pathogenic Wind often serves as the guiding factor of the diseases due to exogenous pathogens, and the ancient doctors thus used pathogenic Wind to summarize all the six exogenous pathogens. This is what is stated in *Gu Kong Lun* (On Spaces of Bones) of *Su Wen* (The Plain Questions): "Wind is the elementary pathogenic factor causing all diseases."

(2) Pathogenic Cold: Cold is the prevalent weather in winter. In winter when the temperature is low, or in the case of sudden decrease of the temperature, man may be affected by Cold if he is not kept in warm.

Diseases caused by pathogenic Cold have two types: affection of Cold and direct attack of Cold. The former refers to a disease due to attack of pathogenic Cold on the superficials of the body which leads to stagnation of the defensive Qi; while the latter refers to direct attack of pathogenic Cold on the Zang Fu organs which often impairs Yang Qi of the Zang Fu organs. Clinically, Cold can be either exogenous or endogenous. The exogenous Cold means attack by the exogenous Cold pathogen; while the endogenous Cold means a morbid condition marked by Deficiency of Yang Qi of the body and the ensuing failure of the Yang Qi to warm the human body. They often affect each other. Patients with endogenous Cold due to Yang Deficiency are more likely to be affected by the exogenous Cold. If exogenous Cold accumulates in the body for a long time, it often impairs Yang Qi of the body to produce the endogenous Cold.

The nature of the pathogenic Cold and the features of the disease caused by Cold are as follows:

① Being a Yin pathogen and liable to impair Yang Qi: Cold is a reflection of exuberance of Yin, so it belongs to Yin. This is so-called that "Excess Yin causing Cold". Yang Qi, as usual, restricts Yin. But when Yin is in Excess, the Yin Cold will violate Yang Qi rather than being expelled by Yang Qi, so it is said that "Excess of

138

Yin impairs Yang". For this reason, affection of Cold pathogen is prone to cause impairment of Yang Qi of the body. When Yang Qi is impaired, it will present Cold manifestations as a result of the deficient Yang failing to perform its warming effect. For example, stagnation of the defensive Qi due to attack of pathogenic Cold on the surface may lead to aversion to cold, direct attack of the pathogenic Cold on the Spleen and the Stomach, impairing the Spleen Yang, often causes cold pain in the epigastric and abdominal region, vomiting, diarrhea, etc. When Cold pathogen attacks Shaoyin (the Heart and the kidney) directly due to Yang Deficiency of both the Heart and the Kidney, there may be such symptoms and signs as aversion to cold, a tendency to lie flat with the limbs huddled up, cold limbs, watery diarrhea with indigested food, profuse clear urine, listlessness and a faint and thready pulse.

② Having the property of stagnating and coagulating: The free flow of Qi, Blood and Body Fluid of the human body completely depends on the warming and propelling of Yang Qi. If Yang is impaired by the excessive Yin, Qi and Blood in the meridians will become stagnated and coagulated as a result of the Cold. So pain often occurs due to obstruction of the Qi and Blood. Thus it is said that Cold is responsible for pain as it has a coagulating and stagnating effect. For example, attack of Cold pathogen on the muscles and skin often obstructs flow of the defensive Qi and the nutritive Qi, leading to headache, pantalgia, etc.

③ Being contracting in nature: This means that Cold pathogen often leads to inward movement of Qi and contraction of the striae of muscles, meridians and vessels, manifested as spasm. For example, attack of pathogenic Cold on the skin and muscles, due to closing of the striae of muscles and inability of the defensive Qi to disperse, may give rise to chills and fever, absence of sweating, etc. When pathogenic Cold attacks vessels, Qi and Blood will become stagnated and the vessels will become convulsive, leading to headache, pantalgia, and tense pulse. And, when pathogenic Cold attack the joints and the meridians, there often appears numbness of the limbs or cold limbs as a result of the convulsion of the meridians.

139

(3) Pathogenic Summer Heat: The Summer Heat, prevalent in summer, is turned from Fire Heat. Diseases caused by Summer Heat are strictly limited to occur in summer, so Summer Heat is a seasonal pathogen. As stated in *Re Lun* (On Heat) of *Su Wen* (The Plain Questions): "Heat pathogen causes febrile disease before the summer solstice, while it causes Summer Heat disease after the summer solstice". Besides, the Summer Heat is always exogenous, so never endogenous Summer Heat is mentioned in TCM.

The nature of pathogenic Summer Heat and the diseases caused by the Summer Heat are as follows:

① Being a Yang pathogen with a hot nature: The Summer Heat is transformed from the Fire Heat in summer. Since Fire Heat is of Yang nature, the Summer Heat belongs to Yang. When Summer Heat invades the human body, it is likely to cause the symptoms marked by Heat such as high fever, dysphoria, red face, and full and large pulse.

② Being dispersive and tending to consume Qi and impair Body Fluid: The Summer Heat is a Yang pathogen which tends to ascend, so the Summer Heat often enters the Qi system directly when it invades the body, leading to opening of the sweat pores and the ensuing profuse sweating. excessive sweating impairs Body Fluid, leading to thirst with preference for drinking, scanty and dark urine, etc. In the case of excessive sweating, Qi will go outwards, following the loss of fluid, thus leading to Deficiency of Qi which is marked by shortness of breath, lassitude, etc. , or even sudden syncope or unconsciousness. If the Summer Heat disturbs the Heart spirit directly, there will be restlessness, chest stuffiness, etc.

③ Often complicated by Dampness: it is not only hot but also wet in summer because it is rainy in this season. As a result of the Heat steaming the Dampness, humidity of the air increases, so Summer Heat often attacks the human body in combination with the Dampness, manifested as the symptoms caused by obstruction of pathogenic Dampness, including incessant fever, difficult sweating, thirst with less intake of water, dirty face, heaviness of the body, lassitude, chest fullness, nausea, vomiting, loose stool or diarrhea.

(4) Pathogenic Dampness: Dampness is the prevalent weather in long-summer which refers to a period between the late summer and the early autumn. In this season, Yang Heat descends to vaporize the Dampness in earth and therefore Dampness spreads in the air. So long-summer is the season with exuberant Dampness in a year. Diseases caused by pathogenic Dampness are either exogenous or endogenous. The exogenous Dampness refers to invasion of the Dampness arising from a wet climate or being caught by rain or living in a damp place; while the endogenous Dampness refers to a morbid state caused by failure of the Spleen to transform and transport water and the resultant retention of Water Dampness in the interior. The exogenous Dampness and the endogenous Dampness often influence each other in the process of disease. Affection of exogenous Dampness often leads to Dampness disturbing the Spleen, causing failure of the Spleen to perform its transforming and transporting function and the resultant production of the endogenous Dampness. On the other hand, Deficiency of the Spleen Yang, which fails to transform water, often causes affection of the exogenous Dampness.

The nature of the Dampness pathogen and the features of the diseases caused by Dampness are as follows:

① Being a Yin pathogen, tending to obstruct flow of Qi and impairing Yang Qi: Dampness is heavy and turbid in nature, similar to water, so it is a Yin pathogen. When retaining in the Zang Fu organs or meridians, pathogenic Dampness often obstructs flow of Qi, leading to disharmony of the ascending and descending movements of Qi and obstruction of meridians, appearing as chest and epigastric distension, dark scanty urine and unsmooth discharge of faeces. As Excess of Yin impairs Yang, invasion of Dampness into the human body is most likely to impair Yang Qi. The Spleen is a Yin organ belonging to earth, serves as the prime organ controlling transformation and transportation of water, likes Dryness and dislikes Dampness, so attack of exogenous pathogenic Dampness disturbs the Spleen first, leading to inhibition of the Spleen Yang and the ensuing failure of the Spleen to transform and transport and retention of water, which is manifested as diarrhea, oliguria, edema or ascites.

② Being heavy and turbid in nature: "Being heavy in nature" means that such symptoms as heaviness of head as if being bound; heaviness of the body and soreness and heaviness of the limbs are often presented in the case of pathogenic Dampness invading the human body. Attack of pathogenic Dampness on the muscles and skin, causing inability of the lucid Yang to ascend and disharmony of the defensive Qi and the nutritive Qi, gives rise to heaviness of the head as if being bound, obstruction of the pathogenic Dampness in the meridians of the joints, leading to obstruction of the distribution of Yang Qi, causes the numbness of the limbs and arthralgia with a heavy sensation. Besides, pathogenic Dampness often presents various kinds of turbid secretions, such as dirty face, lacrimation, sticky loose stool, diarrhea with mucus and blood, humid urine, leukoralgia, excessive exudate in eczema, etc.

③ Being sticky and lingering in nature: This is mainly manifested in two aspects: firstly, Damp disease often presents unsmooth discharge of the sticky secretions and excretions; secondly, disease caused by Dampness, such as eczema and arthralgia due to Dampness, usually has a long course and tends to attack repeatedly.

④ Tending to invade the lower part of the body and the Yin portions of the body: Diseases caused by Dampness exhibit symptoms of the lower parts of the body in most cases. For example, edema is usually more severe in the lower limbs, and such diseases as stranguria, leukorrhea and diarrhea mostly arise from downward flow of pathogenic Dampness. So it is remarked in *Tai Yin Yang Ming Lun* (On the Spleen and the Stomach) of *Su Wen* (The Plain Questions): "When Dampness attacks the human body, it attacks the lower part of the body first".

(5) Pathogenic Dryness: Dryness is the dominant climate in the autumn. In this season, the weather tends to be astringent constantly, thus the air is lack of the moistening of water and becomes dry. Diseases caused by pathogenic Dryness have two types, the warm Dryness and the cool Dryness. In the early autumn, it is still hot, thus Dryness often invades the body together with Heat

pathogen, leading to diseases caused by the Warmth and Dryness. In the later autumn, cold weather of the winter is coming, so the pathogenic Dryness usually invades the human body in combination with the Cold. In most cases, pathogenic Dryness invades the human body through the nose and mouth and tends to attack of the Lung and the superficial part first.

Nature of the pathogenic Dryness and the features of the disease caused by the Dryness are as follows:

① Being dry in nature and tending to impair the Body Fluid: Being dry in nature, pathogenic Dryness is most likely to impair the Body Fluid when it causes diseases, leading to the manifestations of depletion of the Yin Fluid, such as dry mouth and nose, dry throat and thirst, dry hairs, dry or even cracked skin, scanty urine and dry stool. This is so-called Excess of Dryness leading to dry symptoms.

② Impairing the Lung: The Lung is a tender organ which desires for moistening and dislikes Dryness. In addition, the Lung dominates Qi and respiration and connects with the skin and hair, so it is closely related to nature. When pathogenic Dryness invades the human body, it often enters the human body through the mouth and nose or through the skin and the striae of muscles, therefore, pathogenic Dryness tends to impair the Lung Fluid and affect the dispersive and descending effects of the Lung, leading to dry cough without or with little sputum or with mucous sputum which is difficult to be expectorated, dry skin, muscles, mouth and nose, or blood-stained sputum and chest pain with a rushing sensation in the chest.

(6) Pathogenic Fire (Heat): Fire, Heat and Warmth are all caused by Excess of Yang, so they are Heat in nature. As for their difference, Fire arises from the advanced Heat while Heat from the gradual increase of Warmth. Besides, Heat and Warmth are exogenous pathogens in most cases, such as the pathogenic Wind Heat, the pathogenic Warm Heat or the pathogenic Damp Heat, while Fire may present as either the exogenous pathogen or an endogenous pathological state, such as the Heart Fire or the Liver Fire.

The pathogenic Fire as one of the six kinds of exogenous

143

pathogens refers to Heat in fact, so the pathogenic Fire and the pathogenic Heat are often called interchangeably. The main difference between the pathogenic Fire (Heat) and the pathogenic Summer Heat lies in the difference of the corresponding seasons. Usually, diseases caused by Heat pathogen in the summer is considered to be caused by the pathogenic Summer Heat, while those seen in other seasons, by the pathogenic Heat or Warmth itself.

Nature of the pathogenic Fire (Heat) and the features of the diseases caused by the pathogenic Fire (Heat) are as follows:

① Being Yang in nature and having a property of flaring up: Yang stands for motion and going upward. Fire is flammative and goes upward in nature, so it is a Yang pathogen. When impairing the human body, pathogenic Fire (Heat) often causes such symptoms as high fever, aversion to heat, severe thirst, sweating and full and rapid pulse. When such Yang pathogens as Fire or Heat disturb the Heart spirit, they often lead to restlessness, insomnia, mania, coma or delirium. As the Fire tends to flare up, such symptoms as red face and eyes, red tongue tip and margin, erosion in the mouth or the tongue or swollen and painful gums are often detected in diseases caused by Fire.

② Consuming Qi and impairing Body Fluid: Pathogenic Fire (Heat) is most likely to force the Body Fluid to be discharged, impairing Body Fluid and consuming Qi. So, apart from the Heat symptoms, diseases caused by pathogenic Fire (Heat) often produce the symptoms of impairment of the Body Fluid, such as thirst with preference for drinking, dry tongue and throat, scanty and dark urine and constipation. In addition, pathogenic Fire (Heat) tends to consume Qi of the body and thus impairs the Vital Qi, leading to functional decline of the whole body.

③ Tending to cause endogenous Wind and bleeding: Attacking the human body, pathogenic Fire (Heat) is prone to steam in the Liver channel, impairing its Yin Fluid. As a result, the tendons loses the nourishment of the Yin Fluid and endogenous Wind ensues. In this case, a Syndrome, known as extreme Heat producing endogenous Wind will occur, which is marked by high fever, convul-

144

sion, up-staring of the eyeballs, rigidity of the neck, opisthotonus, coma, delirium, etc. When pathogenic Heat enters Blood, they may force Blood to flow swiftly or injure the Blood vessels, leading to various kinds of bleedings, such as haemetemesis, epistaxis, haemefecia, hameturia, macula, menorrhage, metrostaxis and metrorralgia.

④ Causing carbuncle and furuncle: Entering Blood, the pathogenic Fire (Heat) may accumulate in a local area, steaming Blood and muscles to cause carbuncles and furuncles which are manifested as redness, swelling, burning sensation and pain in the affected area, or even ulceration and diabrosis. It is said in *Yi Zong Jin Jian* (A Golden Mirror of Medicine) that "Carbuncles arise from pathogenic toxic Fire."

2. The epidemic exogenous pathogen

The epidemic exogenous pathogen refers to a group of pathogenic factors with strong infectious property. In TCM literature, it is also known as "toxin of infectious disease" or "toxic pathogen". Diseases caused by the epidemic exogenous pathogen are termed *Wen Yi* (infectious disease) or *Yi Li* (fulminating infectious diseases).

Mostly, the epidemic exogenous pathogen invades the human body to cause disease through the nose and mouth, spreading by means of either the air or direct contamination. Diseases caused by the epidemic exogenous pathogen usually possess the following features: ① having sudden onsets and rapid progresses with critical illness condition and similar manifestations; ② being infectious, often causing wide spreading; ③ related to seasonal and climatic conditions; and ④ also related to the environments, diet and sanitary conditions. They may be sporadic or epidemic. Occurrence of epidemic infectious disease is also related to the economic and cultural conditions of society.

3. Internal injury by seven emotions

The seven emotions refer to seven kinds of emotional states, or the joy, the anger, the anxiety, the sorrow, the thinking, the fright and the terror. As the emotional responses of the human body to the stimuli caused by objects, they do not cause diseases in general.

However, when the emotional stimuli are sudden, strong or persistent, they may exceed the adaptive ability of the human body, disturbing flow of Qi and disharmony of Yin, Yang, Qi and Blood of the Zang Fu organs of the body. In this case, they become the pathogenic factors. As they are one of the main pathogens causing internal diseases, they are also known as the seven emotions injuring the interior of the body.

(1) Relations between the seven emotions and Qi and Blood of Zang Fu organs: As a component part of the functional activities of the whole body, the emotional states have a close relationship with Qi and Blood of the Zang Fu organs. Since functional activities of the Zang Fu organs depend on the warming and propelling effects of Qi and the nourishment of Blood, one can carry out his emotional activities only when his Qi and Blood flow freely, his Body Fluid is kept in harmony and his Zang Fu organs function well. For this reason, TCM believes that different emotional states exert different influences on the functional activities of the Zang Fu organs, and the changes of Qi and Blood of the Zang Fu organs, on the other hand, may cause corresponding changes of the emotional states. Therefore, emotional states are closely related to the Qi and Blood of Zang Fu organs. In *Yin Yang Ying Xiang Da Lun* (Manifestations of Yin and Yang) of *Su Wen* (The Plain Questions), it is summarized that the Heart is related to joy in emotions, the Liver to anger, the Spleen to thinking, the Lung to sorrow and the Kidney to terror. Here joy, anger, thinking, sorrow and terror are also called collectively as the five emotions.

(2) Features of disease caused by seven emotions:

① Injuring the internal organs directly: Different from the six exogenous pathogens, the seven emotions cause diseases by injuring the internal organs directly and causing adverse flow of Qi and disharmony between Qi and Blood. Different emotional changes may exert different influence on the different Zang Fu organs, which is summarized in *Yin Yang Ying Xiang Da Lun* (Manifestations of Yin and Yang) of *Su Wen* (The Plain Questions) as joy impairing the Heart, anger impairing the Liver, thinking impairing the Spleen, sorrow impairing the Lung and terror impairing the Kidney.

Clinically, one may not follow this theory mechanically. Man is an organic unity, and the Heart is the master of all the Five Zang organs and the Six Fu organs, so all the emotional stimuli have something to do with the Heart and once the Heart spirit is injured, other Zang Fu organs may also be involved. What is more, as the Heart dominates Blood and houses spirit, the Liver governs free flow of Qi and stores Blood, and the Spleen dominates transformation and transportation, is located in the Middle Jiao and serves as the pivot for ascending and descending movements of Qi as well as the source for generation of Qi and Blood, emotional injury are mostly marked by disturbance of Qi and Blood of these three organs. For example, over-thinking, impairing the Heart and the Spleen, tends to present Deficiency of both Qi and Blood of the Spleen and the Heart, leading to abnormality of the emotional activities and failure of the Spleen to perform its tranforming and transporting effects. In addition, the abnormal emotions tend to tranform into Fire, leading to exuberance of Fire due to Yin Deficiency.

② Affecting flow of Qi in Zang Fu organs: This is an important feature of the seven emotions when they cause disease. In *Ju Tong Lun* (On Examples of Pains) of *Su Wen* (The Plain Questions), this is generalized as anger causing upward adverse flow of Qi, joy causing relaxation of Qi, sorrow causing consumption of Qi, terror causing downward flow of Qi, thinking causing stagnation of Qi and terror causing orderless flow of Qi.

Anger causing upward adverse flow of Qi: Sudden violent rage often causes transverse attack or upward adverse flow of the Liver Qi and the ensuing excessive upward flow of Blood, manifested as red face and eyes, haemetemesis or even sudden syncope with fall.

Joy causing relaxation of Qi: This includes two aspects, relaxing the emotional stress and dismissing the Heart Qi. In normal conditions, joy has the effect of relaxing the emotional stress and promoting flow of the defensive Qi and the nutritive Qi, thus one is kept pleasant. However, overjoy may cause the Heart Qi to be dismissed and the spirit failing to be housed in the Heart, leading to unconcentration or even dementia and mania.

Sorrow causing consumption of Qi: This means that over-sorrow often leads to depression of the Lung Qi, mental depression and consumption of the Lung Qi.

Terror causing sinking of Qi: This indicates that over-sorrow may cause unconsolidation of the Kidney Qi and the ensuing sinking of the Qi, manifested as incontinence of urination and defecation or emission.

Thinking causing stagnation of Qi: Over thinking impairs both the spirit and the Spleen Qi, leading to stagnation of the Spleen Qi. In the case of the stagnation of the Spleen Qi, the Spleen will fail to perform its transforming and transporting function and will cause the ensuing inability of the Stomach to perform its receiving and ripening effects, leading to such symptoms as poor appetite, epigastric and abdominal fullness and loose stool. As a result of the impairment of the Heart Blood, palpitation, insomnia, forgetfulness and dream-disturbed sleep often follow.

③ Emotional changes causing aggravation or sudden deterioration of disease: In the process of disease, if the patients experience violent emotional changes, their conditions may be aggravated or deteriorated suddenly. Heart disease, for example, often becomes aggravated or suddenly deteriorated in the case of emotional changes.

4. Diet, working and resting

Diet, working and resting are the necessary conditions for maintaining the life activities and health. If diet is not regular or limited, or one is in over-working or over-resting, they may disturb the physiological functions of the human body to cause diseases.

(1) Diet as pathogenic factors: Diet should be proper in amount and be taken at regular intervals. Both excessive intake or inadequate intake of food can lead to disease.

① Over eating or over-drinking, or intake of excessive food constantly will exceed the digesting and absorbing ability of the Spleen, causing food retention and impairment of the Spleen and the Stomach, manifested as epigastric and abdominal fullness, eructation and acid regurgitation, anorexia, vomiting and diarrhea. Since the

148

infant's Spleen and Stomach are weaker than the adult's, such diseases affect the infants frequently. Long-term stagnancy of food in the body may transform into Heat, and impairment by cold or cool food may cause accumulation of Dampness and production of Phlegm. In children, long-standing food stagnancy may produce malnutrition, which is manifested as hotness in the palms and soles, dysphoria, irritability, epigastric and abdominal fullness, sallow face and emaciation. Frequent intake of excessive food not only causes indigestion but also affects the flow of Qi and Blood, leading to such diseases as dysentery or haemorrhoid due to stagnation of Blood in the vessels or tendons. If one eats too much fatty or greasy food, he is liable to suffer from interior Heat, causing carbuncles, furuncles, etc.

Failure to eat when hungry or long-standing inadequate intake of food, as a result of inadequate production and supplement of Qi and Blood, will cause insufficiency of Qi and Blood in a chronic case. Deficiency of Qi and Blood, again, causes Deficiency of the Vital Qi and the ensuing decline of the resistant ability against diseases, as a result, other secondary conditions are likely to follow.

② Intake of unclean food: This may causes many kinds of gastrointestinal diseases that are marked by abdominal pain, vomiting, diarrhea, or dysentery, or parasitosis marked by abdominal pain, preference for intake of special things, sallow and emaciation. If one eats rotten or toxic substance, he may present severe abdominal pain complicated by vomiting and diarrhea, or even coma or death in severe cases.

③ Preference for certain food: Intake of too cold or too hot food or preference for food of the certain taste of the five tastes often gives rise to imbalance between Yin and Yang or inadequate intake of some nutritious substances, leading to occurrence of diseases.

Preference for too cold or too hot food: Over intake of raw and cold food may impair the Yang Qi of the Spleen and the Stomach, consequently, Cold Dampness will be generated interiorly, manifested as abdominal pain and diarrhea. In the case of excessive intake of pungent, acrid, warm, dry or hot food, Heat may accumulate in the

149

gastrointestine, leading to thirst, abdominal fullness and pain, constipation or haemorrhoid.

Preference for certain taste of food: All the Qi, Blood and spirit of the human body depend on the five tastes of food for their generation. The five tastes of foods have their own affinity to the Five Zang organs. It is stated in *Zhi Zhen Yao Da Lun* (A Great Treatise on Highlights of Medicine) of *Su Wen* (The Plain Questions) that sour food enters the Liver first, the bitter food enters the Heart first, the sweet food enters the Spleen first, the pungent food enters the Lung first and the salty food enters the Kidney first. If one prefers to the food of one taste only for a long time, the Zang organ corresponding to the taste will become hyperactive, which will impairs the other organs and leads to occurrence of diseases in a chronic conditions. So the foods of different tastes should be taken in combination. In the state of disease, food should be carefully selected. Food that is suitable for the disease may help to treat the disease and promote recovery of the patient from the disease, while that not suitable for the disease may aggravate the disease.

(2) Injury due to over-working or over-resting: Proper working or physical exercise is beneficial to the smooth flow of Qi and Blood and strengthen the constitution. Proper resting, on the other hand, can relieve fatigue, restore one's physical strength and mental activities. However, long-standing over-fitigue or over-resting may become pathogenic factors and cause disease.

① Over fatigue: Over-fatigue includes the following three aspects.

Over physical fatigue: This serves as a pathogenic factor for the disease caused by long-standing over-working. Over physical fatigue impairs Qi, so long-standing over-physical fatigue may cause Deficiency of Qi and reduce of the physical strength which are marked by listlessness and emaciation.

Over mental fatigue: This means that over-thinking may impair the Heart and the Spleen, causing consumption of Heart Blood and impairment of Spleen Qi, which are manifested as the symptoms of malnourishment of the Heart spirit such as palpitation, forgetful-

150

ness, insomnia and dream-disturbed sleep, and the symptoms of failure of the Spleen to transform and transport such as anorexia, abdominal fullness and loose stool.

Intemperance of sexual activities: The Kidney stores essence with storing as its physiological feature. So the Kidney essence must not be excessively discharged. In the case of excessive sexual intercourse, the Kidney essence will be excessively consumed, so such symptoms as soreness and weakness of the loins and knees, dizziness, tinnitus, listlessness, decline of the sexual functions, or nocturnal emission, premature ejaculation or even impotence will occur.

② Over-resting: This indicates that one does not take part in physical working or exercise. Man depends on proper activities to keep free flow of Qi and Blood. If one fails to take part in physical working or exercise for a long time, his Qi and Blood will flow sluggishly, as a result, he will present hypofunction of the Spleen and the Stomach, which is marked by poor appetite, lassitude, listlessness, weakness of the limbs or over-weight, palpitation, shortness of breath and sweating on slight exertion, or other secondary conditions.

In *Xuan Ming Wu Qi Pian* (An Elaboration of the Five Qi) of *Su Wen* (The Plain Questions), diseases caused by over-working or resting are summarized as that prolonged lying impairing Qi, prolonged seeing impairing Blood, prolonged walking impairing tendons, prolonged standing impairing bones, and prolonged sitting impairing muscles.

5. Traumatic injury

Traumatic injury includes the injury caused by gun shot, bombing and knife cut, falls, fractures, contusions and strains, over-loading, burns, freezing and animal or insect bites.

Injuries caused by gun shot, knife cut, falls, contusions and strains, loading and pressing may cause swelling, pain, acchymosis in the affected part or injury of tendons and fracture of bones or dislocations of joints. In severe cases, they may injure the internal organs directly or lead to massive haemorrhage, causing coma, convulsion or death.

Burn often leads to injury of the skin and muscles in mild cases, manifested as redness, swelling, hotness, pain, dryness of skin or blisters with severe pain in the affected parts. In severe cases, it may cause injury of the muscles, tendons and bones and analgesia. The lesion may become feather-like, wax-like, dark yellow in colour or carbonized. In even severe cases with a large affected area, restlessness, fever, thirst, scanty urine or even death often present as a result of severe pain, and vaporization of exudation of Body Fluid apart from the localized symptoms.

Freezing refers to local or systemic injury caused by exposure to lower temperature. Cold is a Yin pathogen and tends to impair Yang Qi. In the case of Excess of Yin Cold, Yang Qi will lose its warming and propelling effects. So freezing of the whole body often presents chills, gradual decrease of the body temperature, pale, purplish colour of the lips, tongue and nails with numbness, lassitude, or drowsiness, feeble breathing, slow and fine pulse, or even death in a chronic course. Local injury often occurs in the hands, feet, ears, tip of the nose and cheeks, which is initially manifested as pale, coldness and numbness of the affected parts, followed by swelling with a blue-purplish colour, itch, pain and hotness, or even blisters of varying sizes. After diabrosis, it tends to produce infections.

Animal and insect injury include bites by animals or lyssodexis, stings by scorpia or bees. In mild cases, it is marked by such symptoms of local injury as swelling, pain or bleeding. In severe cases, it may damage the internal organs or cause death due to massive haemorrhage. Of these injures, bites by snake often causes systemic poisonous symptoms and if not treated promptly, it often causes death. Lyssodexis is marked by local pain and bleeding in its early stage. After healing of the wound in a period of time, it may give rise to restlessness, panic, locked jaw, convulsion, hydrophobia, or windphobia.

6. Phlegm, retained fluid and Blood Stasis

Both Phlegm and retained fluid and Blood Stasis are the pathological products produced in the process of diseases through the action of the pathogenic factors. After their formation, they may directly or indirectly act on the Zang Fu organs or tissues of the body, leading to other secondary diseases, so they are also considered as the pathogenic factors.

(1) Phlegm and retained fluid: Both the Phlegm and the retained fluid are the pathological products formed by disturbance of water metabolism. Generally, Phlegm refers to the thick part while retained fluid, the clear part. Phlegm indicates both the sputum that is expectorated and the Phlegm existing in the Zang Fu organs or in scrofula which is also called invisible Phlegm becasue it is not expectorated from the mouth. The retained fluid is the water retaining in a local area of the human body. It shares different names, depending on the different regions it accumulates. In *Jin Gui Yao Lue* (Synopsis of Prescriptions of the Golden Chamber), the retained fluid is classified as four types, fluid retention in the gastrointestinal tract, pleural effusion, edema and excessive fluid in the hypochondrium.

① Formation of Phlegm and retained fluid: Phlegm and retained fluid mostly arise from disturbance of water metabolism caused by such pathogenic factors as the six exogenous pathogens, improper diet or abnormal emotional changes which destroy the steaming function of the Lung, the Spleen, the Kidney and the Triple Jiao. As the Lung, the Spleen, the Kidney and the Triple Jiao play very important role in water metabolism, functional disturbance of all these organs can lead to formation of Phlegm and retained fluid. After the formation of the Phlegm and the retained food, they will affect the functional activities of the Zang Fu organs, becoming pathogenic factors. Generally speaking, the retained fluid mostly stagnates in the gastrointestinal tract, the pleura and the skin and muscles, while the Phlegm flows with the ascending and descending movements of Qi to reach the Zang Fu organs internally and the skin and muscles externally, leading to multiple diseases, so there is the saying that Phlegm concerns with all diseases.

② Features of diseases caused by Phlegm and retained fluid: After formation, the Phlegm and retained fluid may present different symptoms in the light of the locations of their stagnation. If they stagnate in the meridians, they may affect the flow of Qi and Blood

153

and the functional activities of the meridians; and if they stagnates in Zang Fu organs, they often disturb the functional activities of the Zang Fu organs and the ascending and descending movements of Qi.

Features of the diseases caused by Phlegm: The manifestations of the Phlegm are multifold. In the case of the Phlegm stagnating in the Lung, it may cause dyspnea, cough with sputum. If it stagnates in the Heart, it will cause sluggish flow of Blood which is manifested as chest stuffiness and palpitation. If it confuses the mind, it may cause coma and aphrenia. If it stagnates in the Stomach and leads to adverse flow of the Stomach Qi, it will present nausea, vomiting and epigastric fullness. If it stagnates in the meridians, bones and tendons, it will cause numbness of limbs, hemiplegia or scrofula. If it goes upwards to attack the head, it will give rise to dizziness and syncope. And if it stagnates in the throat, it may cause a feeling of foreign body obstructing in the throat that is difficult to be swallowed or vomited out.

Features of diseases caused by retained fluid: Retained food in the gastrointestinal tract is marked by borborygmus; retention of fluid in the pleura is marked by fullness and pain in the hypochondrium; and overflow of fluid to the skin and muscles is marked by edema, absence of sweat and pain and heaviness of the body.

(2) Blood Stasis: Blood Stasis refers to stagnancy of Blood in the human body, including both the extravasated Blood that fails to be dismissed or the Blood flowing sluggishly or accumulating in the vessels. It is both a pathological product in the process of disease and a pathogenic factor of some diseases.

① Formation of the Blood Stasis: Blood Stasis is caused mainly by two factors:

Deficiency or stagnation of Qi, Blood Cold and Blood Heat often lead to sluiggish flow of Blood and the ensuing occurrence of Blood Stasis. In the case of Qi Deficiency or stagnation of Qi, Blood will fail to be propelled. In the case of Cold attacking Blood, Blood will coagulate. And in the case of Heat entering Blood, the Blood will become stagnated as a result of the sluggish flow of Blood.

Traumatic injury, failure of Qi to control Blood flow or Heat forc-

154

ing Blood to flow swiftly may cause extravasation and the ensuing accumulation of Blood to form Blood Stasis.

② Features of the diseases caused by Blood Stasis: After formation, the congealed Blood will lose its nourishing effect and disturb flow of Blood in a local area or the whole body, producing a series of symptoms. The features of the diseases caused by Blood Stasis vary with the locations and causes of Blood Stasis. If Blood Stasis occurs in the Heart, it will cause palpitation, chest fullness, precardiac pain, purplish colour of the lips and nails. If it occurs in the Lung, it often presents chest pain and coughing blood. If it occurs in the gastrointestinal tract, it may cause haemetemesis and tarry stools. If it occurs in the Liver, it often leads to hypochondriac pain with masses.

Although there are many diseases that are caused by Blood Stasis, their manifestations can be generalized as follows:

Stabbing pain: The stabbing pain is usually fixed, aggravated by pressing and more severe in the night.

Mass or swelling: Traumatic injury to the local area of the skin and muscles often presents blue-purple colour swelling in the affected part. If Blood stagnates in the interior of the body for a long time, abdominal mass which is fixed can be palpated.

Bleeding: The extravasated Blood is usually blue-purple in colour with blood clots.

On observing, there are dark face, squamous and dry skin and muscles, blue purple lips and nails, dark purple tongue or with achymosis and engorgement of the sublingual veins.

Pulse: The pulse is usually fine, uneven, deep wiry or knotted or intermittent.

Mechanism of
Occurrence of Disease

Disease is a concept opposite to health. In TCM, a healthy state is considered to be a state in which the Yin and Yang of the human body are kept in harmony, Qi and Blood flow smoothly and the functional activities of the Zang Fu organs are kept normal. When pathogenic factor acts on the human body, disease will ensue as a result of functional disturbance of the Zang Fu organs and disharmony between Yin and Yang and Qi and Blood.

Although occurrence and changes of disease are rather complicated, they involve both the Vital Qi of the human body and the pathogenic factor at any rate.

1. Occurrence of disease and Vital Qi and pathogen

The Vital Qi refers to the functional activities of the functions of the Zang Fu organs, meridians and the Qi and Blood of the human body, as well as the resistant ability of the human body against disease and the rehabilitating ability of the body. Pathogens refer to various kinds of factors causing diseases. Occurrence and changes of disease are in fact the reflection of the struggles between the Vital Qi and the pathogenic factors.

(1) Deficiency of Vital Qi as the intrinsic basis of occurrence of disease: The theory of occurrence of diseases in TCM put a high value on the Vital Qi of the human body, believing that vicissitude of the Vital Qi determines the occurrence, development and prognosis of a disease. When the Vital Qi is sufficient, which means that the Qi and Blood are sufficient, the functions of the Zang Fu organs are normal and the skin and muscles are well consolidated, pathogen will not be able to enter the human body to cause disease. This is what Ci Fa Lun (On Needling) of Su Wen (The Plain Questions) says: "When Vital Qi is sufficient, pathogens cannot invade." Pathogen can invade the human body by taking advantage of Deficiency of the human body, leading to disharmony between Yin and Yang and the functional disturbance of Zang Fu organs and meridians only when the Vital Qi is relatively deficient, or the skin and muscle are not well consolidated and the resistant ability of the body against disease is weakened. So it is stated in Ping Re Bing Lun (On Febrile Disease) of Su Wen (The Plain Questions) that "Where pathogen attacks, where the Vital Qi is deficient." Therefore, Defi-

ciency of the Vital Qi serves as intrinsic basis of occurrence of disease.

(2) Pathogen as the important precondition for occurrence of disease: Stressing the leading role of the Vital Qi in occurrence of disease, TCM does not exclude the important role of the pathogen in the occurrence of disease, holding that pathogen serves as an important precondition for occurrence of disease or, in given conditions, as the dominant condition. For example, traumatic injury and the epidemic exogenous pathogen may impair or affect the human body once one is exposed to them in spite of his Vital Qi being sufficient. For this reason, it is suggested in *Huang Di Nei Jing* (The Emperor's Internal Classics) that one should keep away from the toxic pathogenic factors to prevent their invasion.

(3) Determination of occurrence of diseases by struggle between the Vital Qi and pathogenic factor: The result of the struggle between the Vital Qi and pathogens determines not only occurrence of disease or not, but also the development and prognosis of a disease.

① Disease that does not occur in the case of Vital Qi winning in the struggle: When pathogen attacks the human body, the Vital Qi will fight against pathogen. If the Vital Qi is strong, pathogen cannot invade the human body, or even it has invaded the human body, it will be eliminated promptly and thus no disease results.

② Disease that occurs in the case of pathogen winning in the struggle: In the process of the struggle between the Vital Qi and the pathogen, if the pathogen is strong and the Vital Qi is relatively deficient, the struggle will result in disturbance of the Qi and Blood and Yin and Yang of Zang Fu organs, and adverse flow of Qi, so disease occurs. After the occurrence of disease, different Syndromes may be presented depending on the difference of the strength of the Vital Qi, the difference of the nature and strength of the pathogens and the difference of the pathogens in depth.

2. Occurrence of disease and the internal and the external environments

The external environment refers to the social and the natural environments. The natural environments include the climatic changes, geographical features and the environmental sanitary conditions, and the social environments indicate the social status, economic condition, the education, the family background, the living experience and the social terms.

(1) Occurrence of disease and the external environments:

① Climatic condition: Different seasons have different common diseases. In the spring, wind is prevalent, so disease caused by Wind Warm are more frequently seen; in the summer, it is hot, so diseases caused by Summer Heat such as febrile disease and heat-stroke are mainly seen in the summer. Occurrence and spreading of infectious disease are also closely related to the climates in nature. When the climatic changes are abnormal, either excessive or deficient, infectious disease are most likely to occur.

② Geographical conditions: Different common diseases are seen in different regions because the natural conditions in different regions are different. As a result of being short of some substances, different endemic diseases may be seen in different regions.

③ Living and working conditions: Living and working conditions also serve as important factors causing diseases. Poor sanitary condition often causes occurrence and spreading of many diseases. Pollution of the environment by waste industrial products or long-term contact of toxic substance may cause poisoning, etc.

In addition, the social environment is also closely related to occurrence of disease.

(2) Occurrence of disease and the internal environment: The internal environment mainly refers to the Vital Qi. As different people have different constitutions, they have different susceptibility to different exogenous pathogens. The strength of the Vital Qi is mainly determined by the constitution and the emotional states.

① Relations between the Vital Qi and the occurrence of disease: Constitution refers to the relatively stable individual difference in both the body physique and the life activities determined by both the congenital factors and the postnatal factors. When the constitution is strong, the functional activities of the Zang Fu organs will be active, and the essence, Qi, Blood and Body Fluid will be sufficient, so disease will not so easily occur. However, when the constitution is weak, the functional activities of the Zang Fu organs will be weakened, and the essence, Qi, Blood and Body Fluid will be insufficient. As a result, the Vital Qi is less strong and disease is likely to occur. The constitution is determined by a number of factors, such as the congenital factors, the feeding, and the physical exercise.

② Relations between the emotional states and the occurrence of disease: TCM puts a high value on the relations between the emotional states and occurrence of disease, which has been clearly described in *Huang Di Nei Jing* (The Yellow Emperor's Internal Classics). It is generally believed that an ease mind with a happy mood can keep Qi flowing freely, and Qi and Blood and the functional activities of the Zang Fu organs in harmony, thus the Vital Qi is sufficient and one is not susceptible to disease. In the case of mental depression, which often leads to adverse flow of Qi, incoordination of Qi, Blood and Yin and Yang, and functional disturbance of the Zang Fu organs, disease is likely to invade the human body. Therefore, maintenance of a proper emotional state can strengthen the Vital Qi, reduce or prevent the occurrence of disease.

Pathogenesis

Pathogenesis refers to the mechanism of occurrence, development and change of disease. Occurrence, development and change of diseases are rather complicated and vary with different diseases and the different manifestations of diseases, but they are related to the constitution and the nature of pathogens as a whole. When pathogen acts on the human body, the Vital Qi will try to ward it off, forming the struggle between the pathogen and the Vital Qi. When pathogen destroys the relative balance between Yin and Yang, leading to functional disturbance of the Zang Fu organs and tissues or Qi and Blood, it will result in various kinds of systemic or local pathological changes. Therefore, rise and decline of the Vital Qi and the pathogen in their struggle, disharmony between Yin and Yang, disturbance of Qi and Blood and functional disturbance of Zang Fu organs form the general law of the changes of the pathogenesis.

Wane and Wax of Pathogen and Vital Qi in Their Struggle

This means changes of the strength of the Vital Qi or the

pathogen in the process of their constant struggle, which not only determines whether occurrence of disease or not, but also determines the Deficiency or Excess of the disease in nature. In addition, it exerts direct influence on the development, change and prognosis of a disease.

1. Wane and wax of pathogen and Vital Qi and the Deficiency or Excess of a disease

In the process of the development and change of a disease, the strengths of the Vital Qi and the pathogen are in constant changes. Generally speaking, increase of the strength of the Vital Qi will give rise to decrease of the pathogen in strength, while the strengthening of the pathogen will impair and consume the Vital Qi. With the wane and wax of the pathogens and the Vital Qi in the human body, disease changes in their Deficiency or Excess nature.

(1) Deficiency or Excess of disease: The pathogenesis of the Deficiency Syndrome or the Excess Syndrome in *Tong Ping Xu Shi Lun* (A General Comment on Deficiency and Excess) of *Su Wen* (The Plain Questions) is summarized as "Excess of pathogen causing Excess Syndrome and Deficiency of Vital Qi causing Deficiency Syndrome".

"Excess" means a morbid state caused mainly by exuberance of pathogen with the Vital Qi not being insufficient, marked by violent struggle between the Vital Qi and the pathogen. As both the Vital Qi and the pathogen are strong, or the pathogen is excessive while the sufficient Vital Qi can resist the pathogen strongly, violent struggle occurs between the Vital Qi and the pathogen, leading to a series of manifestations marked by Excess. In this case, the disease is excessive in nature. The excessive Syndrome is mainly seen in the early or middle stage of an exogenous disease or the Syndrome caused by retention of Phlegm, food, water or Blood in the body. Clinically, Excess Syndrome often presents high fever, mania, high voice, coarse breathing, abdominal pain with tenderness, constipation or retention of urine, and force solid pulse. Besides, accumulation of Phlegm, retention of food, retention of water and stagnation of congealed Blood in the body can all cause the Excess Syndrome.

"Deficiency" is a morbid state mainly caused by Deficiency of the Vital Qi. In other words, it is a pathological reflection of weakness of the Qi, Blood, Body Fluid, Zang Fu organs and meridians and the ensuing failure of the Vital Qi to fight against the pathogen strongly. Therefore, it is usually manifested by Deficiency Syndrome marked by weakness, functional decline and Deficiency of the nutritive substances. The Deficiency Syndrome is mostly detected in the later stage of disease or in patients with weak constitution originally, or in chronic diseases. Such pathological changes as severe or chronic disease consuming the essence Qi, or profuse sweating, severe vomiting and diarrhea or massive bleeding consuming and impairing Qi, Blood, Body Fluid and Yin and Yang of the human body, can all lead to weakness of the Vital Qi, causing such symptoms as listlessness, lassitude, withered face, palpitation, shortness of breath, spontaneous or night sweating, incontinence of urination and defecation, feeble and forceless pulse, or hot sensation over the palms, soles and chest or aversion to cold with cold limbs.

(2) Transformation between Excess and Deficiency and mixture of Excess and Deficiency: Wane and wax of the pathogen and Vital Qi in strength can lead not only to the mere Deficiency or Excess of the Syndrome in nature, but also to transformation of a Syndrome from Excess to Deficiency or vice versa, or the mixture of Deficiency and Excess in a Syndrome.

① Transformation between Deficiency and Excess of Syndrome: This include two aspects: transformation of Excess into Deficiency and that of Deficiency into Excess.

Transformation of Excess into Deficiency: This indicates that an original Excess Syndrome may transform into an Deficiency one due to failure to be treated timely or correctly, due to weakness of the body in senile patients failing to ward off pathogen, or due to consumption of the Qi, Blood and Body Fluid by profuse sweating, severe vomiting, severe diarrhea or massive haemorrhage.

Transformation of Deficiency into Excess: This indicates that a Deficiency Syndrome may transform into an Excess one due to delayed flow or stagnation or metabolic disturbance of the Qi, Blood

162

and Body Fluid and the ensuing accumulation or stagnation of food, Phlegm, retained fluid and Blood Stasis.

② Mixture of Deficiency and Excess: This is a morbid state formed in the process of transformation between Excess and Deficiency Syndrome. For instance, in the process of an Excess Syndrome transforming into a Deficiency Syndrome, Excess of pathogen may coexist with Deficiency of the Vital Qi as a result of the pathogen impairing the Vital Qi. And, in the process of transformation of a Deficiency Syndrome into an Excess one, the Deficiency of the Vital Qi may coexist with the Excess of pathogen as a result of accumulation of the pathological products in the body due to Vital Qi Deficiency.

(3) True or false of Deficiency or Excess: The Deficiency or Excess of pathogenesis must show corresponding symptoms or signs in the clinic. But the symptoms or signs of a disease are only the manifestations. In the case of agreement of the essence of disease with its manifestations, the symptoms or signs can reflect the Deficiency or Excess of the pathogenesis realistically. However, if they are not identical, pseudo manifestations which are not identical with the essence of disease may present. Clinically, a severe Deficiency Syndrome may present pseudo Excess symptoms or signs, while a severe Excess Syndrome may exhibit psudo Deficiency symptoms or signs. True Deficiency Syndrome with pseudo Excess symptoms means that the essence of the disease is deficient with presence of the symptoms of Excess Syndrome, which is mostly caused by failure of the deficient Qi, Blood and Body Fluid to move freely, and true Excess Syndrome with pseudo Deficiency symptoms indicates that the essence of the disease is Excess but with presence of the symptoms of Deficiency Syndrome, which arises mostly from accumulation of excessive pathogen in the interior of the body and the ensuing obstruction of the meridians and inability of Qi and Blood to flow outwards.

2. Wane and wax of pathogen and Vital Qi and the prognosis of a disease

Wane and wax of pathogen and Vital Qi not only determines the

163

Deficiency or Excess of disease but also influence directly the prognosis of disease in its development.

If the Vital Qi wins, pathogen will decrease and thus disease becomes mild or is cured. This is the most commonly seen prognosis of disease, which results from the sufficient Vital Qi fighting against pathogen strongly or from prompt and correct application of treatment. In this case, the pathogen cannot advance further and the pathological impairment of the Zang Fu organs and meridians are repaired gradually, so the Yin and Yang of the body find their balance again on a new basis, and the disease is cured.

In the case of pathogen winning over the Vital Qi in the struggle, disease will progress toward aggravation or cause death, which is mostly caused by Deficiency of the Vital Qi and exuberance of the pathogen leading to constant decline of the resistant ability of the human body against disease, thus the pathogen advances further and the Vital Qi becomes more and more deficient, leading to aggravation of disease. If the Vital Qi is thoroughly exhausted and only the excessive pathogen remains, the life activities of the human body will end and thus death will follow.

In addition, in the case of the strength of the pathogen and that of the Vital Qi being the same, residue pathogen remaining in the body while the Vital Qi being deficient, or failure of the Vital Qi to restore although pathogen have been eliminated, diseases are prone to turn from acute ones to chronic ones or present sequela. This is also the reason for failure of the chronic disease to be cured.

Disharmony
between Yin and Yang

Disharmony between Yin and Yang is a morbid condition marked by Excess or Deficiency of either Yin or Yang, mutual impairment of Yin and Yang, isolation of Yin and Yang and exhaustion of Yin or Yang due to destruction of the balance of Yin and Yang of the human body by some pathogenic factors.

As all the tissues and structures and their functional activities can be classified in accordance with Yin and Yang, disharmony between Yin and Yang can be regarded as a summation of the disharmony between Zang Fu organs, that between meridians, that between Qi and Blood and that between the nutritive Qi and the defensive Qi as well as the incoordination of movements of Qi.

1. Excess of Yin or Yang

This mainly refers to the pathogenesis of the Excess Syndrome marked by Excess of pathogens. Invading the human body, pathogen will act on the Yin or Yang of the body, leading to Excess of Yin or Yang. In the case of Yang pathogen invading the body, Yang of the body will become excessive, while if Yin pathogen invades the body, it will add up Yin to cause Excess of Yin. As Yin and Yang restrict each other, and they are in a state of wane and wax constantly, Yang Excess will restrict Yin, causing its impairment, and Yin Excess will impair Yang, causing its damage.

(1) Excess of Yang: Excess of Yang means exuberance of Yang. It is a morbid state marked by hyperactivity of the human body and excessive heat energy in the human body caused by Excess of Yang in the process of disease. Pathologically, it is characterized by Excess Syndrome of Heat type in which Yang is excessive while Yin is not deficient. In most cases, Yang Excess is caused by affection of warm or Heat pathogens, transformation of Yin pathogens into Heat, Fire transformed from emotional injury, or Heat transformed from stagnation of Qi, Blood Stasis, food retention, etc.

Yang is characterized by heat, motion and dryness, so Yang Excess causes Heat symptoms such as high fever, red face, severe thirst, red eyes, dark urine, dry stools, yellow tongue coating and rapid pulse.

When Yang is excessive, Yin will be relatively deficient, and prolonged Yang Excess will consume Yin Fluid, leading to Yin Fluid Deficiency. So Yang Excess may cause the Syndrome of Yang Heat impairing Yin, and hence there goes the saying that Yang Excess causes disorder of Yin.

(2) Excess of Yin: Excess of Yin, or exuberance of Yin, is a pathological state marked by functional decline or disturbance, insufficiency of heat energy and accumulation of the pathological products in the human body caused by Yin Excess in the process of disease. Usually it is characterized by Excess Syndrome of Cold type in which Yin is excessive while Yang is not deficient. In most cases, Yin Excess is caused by affection of Yin pathogens such as Cold or Dampness, over intake of raw and cold food which leads to obstruction of the Cold and Dampness in the Middle Jiao and inhibition of Yang Qi.

Yin stands for cold, stillness and dampness. So Yin Excess causes cold symptoms, manifested as aversion to cold, cold limbs, abdominal pain with a cold sensation and pale tongue.

When Yin is excessive, Yang will be relatively deficient, and long-standing Yin Excess will impair Yang Qi, leading to decline of Yang and the functional decline of the human body, hence there goes the saying that Yin Excess causes disorder of Yang.

2. Deficiency of Yin or Yang

This refers to the pathogenesis of the Syndromes caused by Deficiency of Vital Qi. Deficiency of the Vital Qi includes the Deficiency of such basic substances of the human body as the essence, Qi, Blood and Body Fluid as well as decline and disharmony of the functions of the Zang Fu organs and meridians. Deficiency of either Yin or Yang will cause its opposite to be relatively excessive due to failure of the deficient side to restrict the other.

(1) Deficiency of Yang: This is a morbid state marked by Deficiency of Yang and the ensuing functional decline or weakness and insufficiency of the heat energy. Pathologically, it is usually characterized by Deficiency syndrome of Cold type in which the Yang Deficiency fails to restrict Yin and thus Yin is relatively hyperactive. In most cases, it is caused by congenital defect, improper feeding after birth, internal injury by over-fatigue or chronic disease in which Yang Qi is impaired.

When Yang Qi is deficient, it will not be able to restrict Yin and

166

its warming effect will decline. As a result, the functional activities of Zang Fu organs and meridians are weakened, Blood and Body Fluid flow sluggishly and water fails to be steamed to produce cold in the interior, which is clinically manifested as pallor and puffy face, aversion to cold with cold limbs, pale tongue, slow pulse, liability to lie flat, listlessness, clear and profuse urine, and diarrhea with indigested food. Generally speaking, Yang Deficiency mainly involves the Spleen and the Kidney, and the Kidney Yang Deficiency, in particular, play an extremely important role in the pathogenesis of Yang Deficiency.

Cold caused by Yang Deficiency and that caused by Yin Excess are different in both pathogenesis and clinical manifestations. The former is marked by Deficiency complicated with Cold, while the latter, by Cold without evident Deficiency.

(2) Deficiency of Yin: This is a morbid state marked by Deficiency of such Yin Fluids of the body as the essence, Blood and Body Fluid, failure of Yin to restrict Yang and the ensuing hyperactivity of Yang, and the hyperfunction of the body of Deficiency type. Usually it causes a Deficiency Syndrome of Heat type marked by Deficiency of Yin Fluid, decline of the nourishing and calming effects of Yin and the resultant hyperactivity of Yang. This condition is mainly due to impairment of Yin by Yang pathogens, impairment of Yin by the Fire transformed from emotional disturbance or consumption of Yin in a chronic disease.

Different Syndromes such as interior Heat due to Yin Deficiency, flaring up of Fire due to Yin Deficiency and hyperactivity of Yang due to Yin Deficiency may follow Deficiency of Yin as a result of inability of Yin to restrict Yang. Clinically, interior Heat due to Yin Deficiency is mainly marked by hotness sensation over the palms, soles and chest, bone Heat, tidal fever, flushing of face, night sweating, emaciation, dry mouth and throat, red tongue with little coating and fine and rapid pulse. It mainly involves the Kidney Yin and the Liver Yin, especially the Kidney Yin which plays an extremely important role in the pathogenesis of Yin Deficiency.

Heat due to Yin Deficiency is also different from Heat due to Yang

Excess in both pathogenesis and clinical manifestations. The former is marked by Deficiency complicated by Heat, while the latter is mainly marked by Heat without evident Deficiency.

3. Mutual impairment of Yin and Yang

On the basis of Yin Deficiency or Yang Deficiency, if Deficiency of the both occurs as a result of Yin or Yang Deficiency affecting its opposite, it is known as mutual impairment of Yin and Yang. As the Kidney stores essence Qi, houses the genuine Yin and the genuine Yang which serve as the basis of Yin and Yang of the whole body, both Yin Deficiency and Yang Deficiency can affect its opposite only when they damage the essence Qi of the Kidney or they are the Deficiency of the Kidney Yin or Kidney Yang.

(1) Yin Deficiency affecting Yang: This is a morbid state marked by Deficiency of both Yin and Yang with Yin Deficiency as the main aspect caused by Yin Deficiency leading to inadequate production of Yang Qi or failure of Yang Qi to be attached to Yin based on Yin Deficiency. Rising of the Liver yang, which is commonly seen in the clinic, for example, is originally a Syndrome characterized by Deficiency of the Kidney water and the ensuing failure of the Kidney water to restrict the Liver Yang. With the further development of the disease, the Kidney essence may be impaired, so Kidney Yang Deficiency, marked by aversion to cold, cold limbs, pale and puffy face, deep weak pulse and pale tongue, develops based on the Kidney Yin Deficiency and as a result, Yin Deficiency affecting Yang follows.

(2) Yang Deficiency affecting Yin: This is a morbid state marked by Deficiency of both Yin and Yang with Yang Deficiency as the main aspect developed based on Yang Deficiency which leads to failure of Yin to be adequately generated. For example, edema, a commonly seen symptom in the clinic, is usually caused by insufficiency of Yang which fails to steam water and thus water retains in the body or flows over to the skin and muscles. With the further development of the disease, Yin will fail to be generated by Yang and become more and more insufficient, as a result, such symptoms of Yin Deficiency as emaciation, restlessness, or even tremor will present, leading to the Syndrome of Deficiency of both Yin and Yang with

Yang Deficiency as the main aspect.

4. Isolation of Yin and Yang

This includes two types, Yang being kept in the exterior by excessive Yin and Yin being kept in the exterior by excessive Yang. Both of them are caused by accumulation of extremely strong Yin or Yang in the interior which keeps its opposite to stay in the exterior and the ensuing incoordination between Yin and Yang. Clinically, they give rise to such complicated pathological changes as true Cold complicated with pseudo Heat manifestations and true Heat complicate with pseudo Cold manifestations.

(1) Yang being kept in the exterior by excessive Yin: This is a morbid state marked by isolation of Yin from Yang due to accumulation of excessive Yin in the interior which forces Yang to stay in the exterior and the ensuing incoordination between Yin and Yang. The essence of the disease lies in Yin Excess in the interior, but as the Yang is kept in the exterior, there are such pseudo manifestations as red face, restlessness, thirst, preference to take away quilt or coats, mania and large pulse. In this case, it causes the Syndrome of true Cold complicated by pseudo Heat manifestations.

(2) Yin being kept in the exterior by excessive Yang: This is a morbid state marked by failure of Yang Qi to reach the limbs due to accumulation of pathogenic Heat in the interior. The essence of the disease lies in accumulation of excessive Yang in the interior, but as Yin is kept in the exterior, there are such pseudo Cold manifestations in the clinic as cold limbs and deep or hidden pulse. In this case, it causes the Syndrome of true Heat complicated by pseudo Cold manifestations.

5. Exhaustion of Yin or Yang

Exhaustion of Yin and Yang, including exhaustion of Yin and exhaustion of Yang, is a morbid state marked by sudden and severe loss of Yin Fluid or Yang Qi of the body and the ensuing exhaustion of the functional activities of the human body.

(1) Exhaustion of Yin: This is a morbid state marked by sudden loss of Yin Fluid of the human body which leads to exhaustion of the functional activities of the human body. It is mostly caused by se-

vere impairment of the Yin Fluid by exuberant pathogenic Heat or lingering of the pathogenic Heat or by other pathogenic factors. Clinically, it is manifested as constant perspiration, hot and sticky sweat, warm limbs or even coma, delirium and rapid but forceless pulse.

(2) Exhaustion of Yang: This is a morbid state marked by sudden severe loss of Yang Qi of the body and the ensuing exhaustion of the functional activities of the human body. It is usually caused by exuberant pathogen winning the victory in the struggle between Yang Qi and the pathogen, over-fatigue in patients with original Yang Deficiency, over-use of diaphoresics which leads to excessive sweating and the resultant excessive discharge of Yang Qi following the sweating, or impairment of Yang Qi in a chronic disease developing exhaustion of Yang Qi. Clinically it is manifested as profuse sweating with the sweat being cold and clear, cold limbs, cold skin, listlessness, dull complexion, or even coma and feeble and indistinct pulse.

As Yin and Yang depend on each other and assist each other, exhaustion of Yang often follows in the case of Yin exhaustion as a result of the Yang failing to attach to Yin and the ensuing outward floating of Yang. In the case of Yang exhaustion, Yin will also be exhausted because it is not generated adequately. So exhaustion of both Yin and Yang or death often results in the case of exhaustion of Yin or Yang.

Disturbance of Qi and Blood

This includes the pathological changes caused by disturbance of Qi in amount and function, that of Blood in amount and function, and that of the mutual dependence and mutual assistance relationships between Qi and Blood.

1. Disturbance of Qi

This includes two aspects: Qi Deficiency which is caused by inadequate production or excessive consumption of Qi and decline of the functions of Qi, and disturbance of Qi in movements.

(1) Qi Deficiency: This is a morbid state marked by consumption of the genuine Qi and the functional decline of Qi which leads to decline of the functions of Zang Fu organs and lowering of the resistant ability against disease. Qi Deficiency includes Deficiency of such Qi as the genuine Qi, the pectorial Qi, the defensive Qi and the nutritive Qi, and the decline of the propelling, warming, defending, controlling and steaming effects of Qi. In most cases, Qi Deficiency is caused by congenital defect, improper feeding after birth, consumption of Qi by over-fatigue, failure of Qi to restore in a protracted disease, or inadequate production of Qi due to functional disturbance of the Lung, the Spleen and the Kidney. Clinically, it is usually manifested as listlessness, lassitude, dizziness, spontaneous sweating, weak pulse, liability to suffer from cold, etc.

(2) Disturbance of Qi in movements: This refers to the pathological changes marked by stagnation of Qi, upward adverse flow of Qi, collapse of Qi, obstruction of Qi and escape of Qi due to disturbance of the ascending, descending, out-going and entering movements of Qi.

Ascending, descending, out-going and entering, the basic patterns of Qi's movement, are the fundamental process of the functional activities of the Zang Fu organs, meridians, Qi and Blood, and Yin and Yang. They determines the functional activities of the Zang Fu organs and meridians, the harmony and balance between the Zang Fu organs and meridians, Qi and Blood and Yin and Yang. Therefore, disturbance of Qi in movements involves various kinds of diseases concerning the Five Zang organs, the Six Fu organs, the exterior and interior of the body, the four limbs and the nine orifices of the human body. Clinically, disturbance of Qi in movements can be generalized as the following patterns.

① Stagnation of Qi: This is mostly caused by emotional depression, exposure to cold, or obstruction of Phlegm, Dampness, retained food and Blood Stasis which obstruct flow of Qi, causing stagnation of Qi in the whole body or in a local area and the ensuing

171

functional disturbance of some Zang Fu organs and meridians. Stagnation of Qi in a local area often leads to a feeling of fullness and distension and pain in the area. If the stagnation of Qi affects flow of Blood or Body Fluid, it may cause such pathological products as Blood Stasis, Phlegm and retained fluid. Besides, stagnation of Qi can also lead to functional disturbance of some Zang Fu organs, such as accumulation of the Lung Qi, stagnation of the Liver Qi, and stagnation of Qi in the Spleen and Stomach.

② Upward adverse flow of Qi: This is a morbid state marked by upward adverse flow of Qi of Zang Fu organs arising from disturbance of the ascending and descending movements of Qi, which is mostly caused by emotional injury, improper diet, or obstruction of Phlegm. It involves the Liver, the Stomach and the Lung in most cases. When Lung Qi fails to descend and goes upward, cough will result. If the Stomach Qi runs upward, it will cause nausea, vomiting, hiccup, or eructation. When the Liver Qi rises excessively, it will cause headache with a distending sensation, fullness and distention in the hypochondriac region, red face and eyes, and irritability, or even haemetemesis, coughing blood or syncope in the case of Blood rushing upward following the Liver Qi.

Upward adverse flow of Qi is mostly seen in Excess Syndrome, but it may also be found in the Deficiency one. For example, the Lung Qi may go upward if the deficient Lung Qi fails to move downward or when the Kidney Qi fails to receive the fresh air; failure of the Stomach Qi to descend in the case of Stomach Qi Deficiency may cause upward adverse flow of the Stomach Qi, etc.

③ Collapse of Qi: This refers to a morbid state marked by the deficient Qi failing to lift, which is mostly caused by the further development of Qi Deficiency. The relative fixation of the positions of Zang Fu organs in the human body depends on the ascending, descending, out-going and entering movements of Qi. If Qi fails to lift due to Deficiency, prolapse of visceral organs, such as gastroptosis, nephroptosia, and prolapse of uterus, will ensue as a result. As the Spleen and the Stomach serve as the source for generating Qi and Blood, Qi collapse is most likely to occur in the case of Deficiency of the Spleen Qi or the Stomach Qi. So collapse of Qi of the Middle Jiao (including the Spleen and Stomach) is the mostly commonly seen type of collapse of Qi, which is marked by fullness with a lowering down sensation in the abdomen and lumbar region, frequent occurrence of desires for defecation, shortness of breath, lassitude, lower voice, and weak pulse.

④ Obstruction of Qi and escape of Qi: Both of the obstruction of Qi and the escape of Qi are the morbid states marked by disturbance of the entering and out-going movements of Qi, which are clinically manifested as syncope or prostration in the clinic.

Obstruction of Qi: This is mostly caused by obstruction of turbid pathogen on the exterior of the human body or severe stagnation of Qi in the interior, which leads to failure of Qi to go outward and the clear orifice (the brain) to be well supported. As a result, syncope of obstructing type, which is marked by cold limbs and coma, follows.

Escape of Qi: This is mostly caused by sudden impairment of the Vital Qi by strong pathogens, or the constant aggravation of Vital Qi Deficiency leading to outward escape of the Vital Qi, or by massive haemorrhage or profuse sweating which leads to excessive discharge of Qi. As a result of escape of Qi, the functional activities of the human body present sudden exhaustion.

2. Disturbance of Blood

Disturbance of Blood consists of two aspects: Deficiency of Blood which arises from inadequate production of Blood, excessive consumption of Blood or decline of the nourishing effect of Blood; and disturbance of Blood in circulation, including sluggish flow of Blood, swift flow of Blood, or the adverse flow of Blood which often leads to Blood Stasis, Blood Heat and bleeding.

(1) Blood Deficiency: This is a morbid state marked by insufficiency of Blood in volume or decline of the nourishing effects of Blood, mostly caused by excessive loss of Blood, Deficiency of the Spleen and Stomach or inadeqaute intake of nutrients which leads to decline of the function of generating Blood and the ensuing inadequate production of Blood, or consumption of Blood in a lingering

173

disease and consumptive disease.

All the Zang Fu organs and tissues of the human body depend on the nourishment of Blood, so Blood Deficiency will give rise to malnutrition of the whole body or a part of the body, leading to decline of the functional activities, manifested as lustreless face, pale lips, tongue and nails, dizziness, vertigo, palpitation, listlessness, lassitude, emaciation, or numbness of the limbs, inability of the limbs to extend or flex freely, or dry eyes and blurred vision.

(2) Blood Stasis: This is a morbid state marked by sluggish or delayed flow of Blood, which is mostly caused by the stagnated Qi obstructing flow of Blood, the deficient Qi failing to move Blood, obstruction of Phlegm in the vessels, invasion of pathogenic Cold into vessels which causes coagulation of Blood, or invasion of pathogenic Heat into vessels which steams the Body Fluid in the Blood. The main pathogenesis of Blood Stasis lies in that the Blood flows sluggishly or even coagulates to form the Blood Stasis, which, again, obstructs in the vessels to become another factor causing Blood Stasis. Obstruction of Blood in a local area, including the Zang Fu organs or meridians, will present fixed pain which is not relieved by warmth or cold, or even masses, complicated by dark face, squamous and dry skin and muscles, dark purple colour of the lips and tongue with or without acchymosis, etc.

Blood Stasis may also aggravate stagnation of Qi, leading to a vicious cycle in which the stagnation of Qi causes Blood Stasis and the Blood Stasis aggravates the stagnation of Qi.

(3) Blood Heat: This is a morbid condition marked by invasion of pathogenic Heat into Blood and the ensuing acceleration of Blood flow, which is mostly caused by invasion of pathogenic Heat into Blood, or Fire transformed from emotional upsets. Blood Heat will force Blood to flow swiftly, or even injure the vessels to cause bleeding. Besides, it may also steam and consume the Blood and Body Fluid. So, the symptoms caused by Blood Heat include the symptoms of Heat, the symptoms of consumption of Blood, the symptoms of extravasation and the symptoms of impairment of Yin Fluid, such as fever which is more severe at night, dry mouth but

without desire for drinking, dysphoria, mania, or epistaxis, haemetemesis, haematuria, preceded menstruation or menorrhagia, red or
dark red tongue and fine and rapid pulse.

3. Disturbance of the relations between Qi and Blood

Qi belongs to Yang and Blood to Yin, so Qi and Blood depend upon each other and assist each other. Disturbance of ascending, descending, out-going and entering movements of Qi will affect the
Blood at any rate, while depletion of Blood or its functional disturbance of Blood, or the other way round, will affect Qi. Clinically,
the commonly seen incoordination between Qi and Blood are as follows:

(1) Stagnation of Qi and Blood Stasis: This is a morbid state
marked by unsmooth flow of Qi which leads to disturbance of Blood
flow and the resultant Blood Stasis, which arises from emotional depression that causes stagnation of Qi and Blood Stasis, or from fall,
contusion, etc. which causes concurrence of stagnation of Qi and
Blood Stasis. Clinically, it is usually manifested as distending pain,
petechia or masses. In addition, this morbid state is closely related
to the functional disturbance of the Liver and the Heart.

(2) Failure of Qi to control Blood: This is a morbid state marked
by various kinds of bleedings such as coughing blood, epistaxis,
haemetemesis, haemefecia, hameturia or metrostaxis and metror-
rhagie, caused by the deficient Qi failing to perform its controlling
effect on Blood flow and the ensuing occurrence of extravasation. Of
the bleedings, bleeding in the lower part of the body due to collapse
of the deficient Qi is most commonly seen.

(3) Deficiency of both Qi and Blood: This is a morbid state
marked by coexistence of both Qi Deficiency and Blood Deficiency,
which is usually caused by impairment of Qi and Blood in chronic
disease, Deficiency of Qi following Deficiency of Blood, Deficiency
of Blood following Deficiency of Qi as a result of the deficient Qi
failing to generate Blood, etc. Clinically, it is manifested as pale or
sallow complexion, shortness of breath, disinclination to talk, lassitude, loss of weight, palpitation, insomnia, dry skin and numbness
of limbs.

175

In addition, such Syndromes as escape of Qi following haemorrhage and inability of Qi and Blood to nourish meridians are also commonly seen in the clinic.

Disturbance of Body Fluid Metabolism

The normal metabolism of Body Fluid not only maintains the harmonious balance among the formation, distribution and discharge of Body Fluid, but also serves as an important precondition for the performance of the physiological functions of Zang Fu organs of the human body. Therefore, disturbance of Body Fluid metabolism will cause a series of disturbance of the physiological functions of the human body.

1. Insufficiency of the Body Fluid

This is a morbid state marked by reduce of the Body Fluid in amount and the ensuing loss of moistening of the Zang Fu organs, skin and orifices of the human body with presence of the symptoms of dryness, which is mostly caused by affection of pathogenic Dryness, impairment of Body Fluid by the Fire transformed from emotional upsets, or consumption of Body Fluid due to fever, profuse sweating, vomiting, diarrhea, profuse urine, haemorrhage or over use of pungent and dry drugs.

Jin (the clear part of Body Fluid) and Ye (the thick part of the Body Fluid) are somewhat different in their nature, distribution and physiological functions, so manifestations of impairment of Jin are also somewhat different from those of consumption of Ye. Generally, such manifestations as profuse sweating in hot summer; thirst with preference for drinking in high fever, dry skin, mouth and nose in dry weather; and sinking of eyes, and systremma caused by severe vomiting, diarrhea or profuse urine are considered to be the impairment of Jin, while the smooth tongue with little or without coating, dry mouth and tongue without a desire for drinking, emacia-tion, withering of the skin and hairs seen in the later stage of febrile disease or in Deficiency of essence and Blood caused by chronic disease are considered to be the manifestations of consumption of Ye.

In most cases, consumption of Ye may not be complicated in the case of impairment of Jin. However, impairment of Jin must be complicated in the case of consumption of Ye. For this reason, Jin is more easily impaired and supplemented than Ye, and although Ye is not so easily consumed, it is also difficult to be supplemented immediately once it is consumed.

2. Disturbance of Body Fluid in distribution and discharge

Distribution and discharge of Body Fluid are two important links in the metabolism of Body Fluid. Disturbance of distribution of Body Fluid is different from that of the discharge of Body Fluid, but both of them can result in retention of Body Fluid in the human body, producing such pathological products as Dampness, Phlegm, retained fluid and edema.

Disturbance of Body Fluid in distribution refers to failure of the Body Fluid to be distributed normally and the ensuing delayed flow of the Body Fluid in the human body or its retention in a local area. As a result, Body Fluid is not timely steamed and Dampness, Phlegm or retained fluid is produced. The main reasons for disturbance of Body Fluid in distribution include failure of the Lung Qi to perform its dispersing and descending effects, inability of the Spleen to transform and transport, stagnation of the Liver Qi and dysfunction of the Triple Jiao as the water passageway. Of these reasons, failure of the Spleen to transform and transport is the most important, so it is said in *Zhi Zhen Yao Da Lun* (A Great Treatise on Highlights of Medicine) in *Su Wen* (The Plain Questions) that "Diseases marked by fullness and edema due to Dampness are ascribed to the Spleen in most cases."

Disturbance of Body Fluid in discharge mainly refers to decline of the function of the Body Fluid to be transformed into sweat or urine, which leads to retention of water and the ensuing edema due

177

to over-flow of water. Transformation of Body Fluid into sweat mainly depends on the dispersive effect of the Lung Qi, while that into urine on the steaming effect of the Kidney. Thus, functional decline of the Kidney and the Lung, especially that of the Kidney, serves as the main cause of retention of water.

Disturbance of the distribution and discharge of Body Fluid often influence each other, leading to generation of water, retained fluid, Phlegm and Dampness in the interior and the ensuing development of a number of diseases.

3. Disturbance of the relations between Body Fluid and Qi or Blood

Coordination of the functions of the Body Fluid and Qi and Blood is an important factor contributing to the normal performance of the physiological activities of the human body. If this relationship is disturbed, various kinds of diseases will ensue as a result.

(1) Retention of water and obstruction of Qi: This mainly refers to a morbid state marked by disturbance of water metabolism which causes retention of water, Phlegm or Dampness and the ensuing obstruction of flow of Qi. For example, retention of fluid in the Lung can lead to accumulation of the Lung Qi, causing disturbance of the dispersive and the descending function of the Lung, which is manifested as chest fullness, cough, and asthma with inability to lie flat. When water attacks the Heart, it may obstruct the Heart Qi or the Heart Yang, causing palpitation and cardiac pain.

(2) Depletion of Body Fluid and Dryness of Blood: This mainly refers to a morbid state in which depletion of Body Fluid leads to Blood Dryness and generation of Heat of Deficiency type or Blood Dryness and generation of the endogenous Wind. Body Fluid and Blood are derived from the same source, and the Body Fluid is an important component part of the Blood. Depletion of Body Fluid and Blood Dryness will occur in the case of high fever impairing Body Fluid, burns causing depletion of Body Fluid, haemorrhage leading to consumption of Body Fluid or impairment of Body Fluid by Heat produced by Yin Deficiency. Clinically, it is usually manifested as restlessness, dry nose and throat, hotness sensation over the

178

palms, soles and chest, emaciation, scanty dark urine, red tongue with little coating, fine and rapid pulse, or dark skin or even squamous and dry skin, itching or desquamation.

Besides, such morbid states as escape of Qi following excessive discharge of Body Fluid and Blood Stasis caused by depletion of Body Fluid are also commonly seen in the clinic.

The Five Kinds of
Endogenous "Pathogens"

This refers to five kinds of morbid states manifestations of which are similar to those of the diseases caused by attack of the exogenous Wind, exogenous Cold, exogenous Dampness, exogenous Dryness and exogenous Fire, due to disturbance of the functional activities of Qi, Blood, Body Fluid and the Zang Fu organs in the process of disease. As they are not caused by attack of exogenous pathogens, they are so called. In other words, the five kinds of endogenous "pathogens" are in fact the five kinds of pathogeneses instead of five pathogens.

1. The endogenous Wind

The endogenous Wind is a morbid condition caused by hyperactivity of Yang Qi of the human body. As it is closely related to the Liver, it is also known as stirring of the Liver Wind or just briefly as the Liver Wind. Excessive ascending of Yang Qi, either due to exuberance of Yang or due to Deficiency of Yin which fails to restrict Yang, may cause the endogenous Wind if it gives rise to such symptoms as shaking, dizziness, convulsion and tremor in the process of disease. Clinically, the commonly encountered endogenous Wind can be classified as the following types.

(1) Extreme Heat producing Fire: This is mainly seen in the advanced stage of febrile disease in which the exuberant pathogenic Heat impairs the Body Fluid or the Ying Blood and burns the Liver

179

channel, leading to loss of nourishment of tendons and hyperactivity of Yang and the ensuing occurrence of the endogenous Wind. Wind produces symptoms of motility, so there are convulsion, tremor, rigidity of neck, opisthotomus, up-staring of the eyeballs, complicated by high fever, coma or delirium.

(2) The Liver Yang transforming into Wind: This is mostly caused by impairment of the Liver Yin and the Kidney Yin due to emotional injury or over-fatigue, which leads to Yin being unable to restrict Yang and the ensuing hyperactivity or excessive rising of Yang, which, in a chronic case, will cause more severe depletion of Yin and more severe floating of Yang and the final occurrence of the endogenous Wind as a result of hyperactivities of the Liver Yang. Clinically, it is manifested as muscular twitching and cramp, numbness and tremor of limbs, dizziness with a tendency to fall, or distortion of the mouth and eyes or hemiplegia in a mild case, or as sudden fall, syncope of obstructing type or prostration in severe cases.

(3) Yin Deficiency producing Wind: This is mostly seen in the later stage of febrile diseases in which the Yin is depleted or consumed by the protracted disease. As a result of Yin depletion, tendons lose nourishment and thus endogenous Wind follows. So this is an endogenous Wind of Deficiency type. Clinically it is manifested as convulsion, muscular twitching and cramp, involuntary movement of the limbs and the symptoms of interior Heat due to Yin Deficiency.

(4) Blood Deficiency producing Wind: This is usually caused by inadequate production or excessive lose of Blood which leads to malnutrition of the tendons or failure of Blood to nourish vessels and the ensuing generation of the endogenous Wind. Clinically it is manifested as numbness of limbs, muscular twitching and cramp, or even convulsion or inability of the limbs to flex and extend.

(5) Blood Dryness producing Wind: This is mostly caused by impairment of Yin and consumption of Blood by protracted disease, depletion of essence and Blood in the aged, long-standing inadequate intake of nutrients or Blood Stasis which leads to disturbance of gen-

eration of Blood. In the case of depletion of Body Fluid and Blood Deficiency, Dryness will ensue as a result. So, the muscles and skin loss the nourishment and Qi and Blood in the meridians lose their harmony, leading to endogenous Wind. Clinically, it is mainly manifested as dry skin, itching or desquamation or squamous and dry skin.

2. The endogenous Cold

This is a morbid state marked by generation of Cold of Deficiency type in the interior or dispersion of the Yin Cold pathogen in the interior caused by Deficiency of Yang Qi and the ensuing decline of its warming and steaming effects.

Failure of the deficient Kidney Yang and the deficient Spleen Yang to perform their warming and steaming effects are the main reasons for the endogenous Cold. The pathogenesis of the endogenous Cold lies in two aspects: Yin Excess due to failure of the deficient Yang to restrict Yin and the ensuing production of the endogenous Cold, which is characterized by aversion to cold, cold limbs, pale complexion, inclination to lie flat, desire for warmth, diarrhea with loose stools, moist tongue coating and no thirst and retention or accumulation of such pathological products of Yin nature as water, retained fluid and Phlegm due to Yang Deficiency and decline of its steaming effect, which is marked by frequent, profuse and watery urine, discharge of thin, cold and clear saliva, sputum and nasal discharge, diarrhea or edema.

The endogenous Cold is both different from and connected with the exogenous Cold. The endogenous Cold is marked by both Deficiency and Cold with Deficiency as the main aspect, while the exogenous Cold is only marked by Cold. Attacking the human body, the exogenous Cold is liable to impair Yang Qi and may finally lead to Yang Deficiency, while a patient with original Yang Deficiency, is most likely to suffer from the disease caused by invasion of the exogenous pathogen.

3. The endogenous Dampness

This is a morbid state marked by accumulation or retention of water, Dampness or Phlegm due to decline or disturbance of the

Spleen's transforming and transporting effects. As it is mostly caused by Spleen Deficiency, it is also known as Spleen Deficiency producing Dampness.

Generation of endogenous Dampness is usually caused by overweight with excessive Phlegm or Dampness, over-intake of raw and cold food or greasy and fatty food impairing the Spleen and the Stomach which leads to failure of the Spleen to transform and transport, disturbance of water metabolism, failure of water to be transformed and the ensuing production of Dampness, Phlegm, retained fluid or edema. Failure of the Spleen to transform and transport is the main factor contributing to formation of the endogenous Dampness, and the transforming and transporting effects of the Spleen depend on the warming and steaming effects of the Kidney Yang, so formation of the endogenous Dampness is also closely related to the Kidney.

The clinical manifestations of the endogenous Dampness vary with the different positions the Dampness obstructs. Retention of Dampness in the meridians often presents a heavy sensation in the head as if being bound, and heavy sensation in the limbs with inability of the limbs to flex or extend. Attack of Dampness on the Upper Jiao often causes chest distention with cough. Obstruction of Dampness in the Middle Jiao often leads to fullness and distention in the epigastric region or abdomen, poor appetite, sticky or sweet taste in the mouth, and thick and greasy tongue coating. Retention of Dampness in the Lower Jiao is usually manifested as abdominal distention, loose stools and oliguria. And overflow of Dampness to the skin and muscles will cause edema. Of these pathological changes, obstruction of Dampness in the Middle Jiao is a Syndrome always seen in diseases caused by the Dampness.

The endogenous Dampness and the exogenous Dampness affect each other. When exogenous Dampness invades the body, it is prone to impair the Spleen, leading to failure of the Spleen to transform and transport and the resultant production of the endogenous Dampness. On the other hand, a patient with original exuberance of Dampness is likely to suffer from the disease caused by invasion of

182

exogenous Dampness.

4. The endogenous Dryness

This is a morbid condition marked by Dryness due to the deficient Body Fluid failing to moisten organs, tissues and orifices.

The endogenous Dryness is mostly caused by impairment of Yin Fluid in chronic disease, impairment of Yin by Heat pathogen, consumption of Yin Fluid by over-use of diaphoresics, severe vomiting and diarrhea, loss of Blood or essence, or by the Dryness transformed from Dampness. As a result, consumption of the Body Fluid leads to production of Dryness Heat, and that the manifestations of Dryness occur.

Clinically, endogenous Dryness may be caused by either depletion of Yin Fluid or excessive pathogenic Heat impairing Body Fluid, and although it may be seen in all the organs and tissues of the human body, it affects the Lung, the Stomach and the Large Intestine most frequently. The endogenous Dryness is marked by Dry Heat symptoms, such as dry and lustreless skin, desquamation or even cracked skin, dry mouth and throat, dry lips, absence of fluid on the tongue coating or smooth tongue with fissures, dry cough without sputum, fragile nails, dry stools and scanty dark urine.

5. The endogenous Fire (Heat)

This is a morbid state marked by functional hyperactivity of the human body and generation of Fire in the interior arising from excessive Yang, hyperactivity of Yang due to Yin Deficiency, stagnation of Qi and Blood and accumulation of pathogens.

The pathogeneses of endogenous Fire or Heat can be classified as Fire transformed from excessive Yang, that transformed from stagnated pathogen, that transformed from emotional stress and that caused by Yin Deficiency. And as a whole, it can be divided into two types, the Excess and the Deficiency. The excessive Fire arises mostly from Excess of Yang or stagnation of pathogen transforming into Fire, with a rapid progression and a short course. Clinically it is manifested as high fever, red face, thirst with desire for cold drinking, dark urine, constipation, ulcer or erosion in the mouth or tongue, red tongue, red eyes, yellow and dry tongue coating, full and rapid pulse, or even coma and mania. The deficient Fire is mostly caused by hyperactivity of Yang due to depletion of essence and Blood and the ensuing up-flaring of Fire of the Deficiency type, with a slow progression and a long disease course. Clinically it is usually manifested as hot sensation in the soles, palms and chest, bone Heat, tidal fever, red cheeks in the afternoon, insomnia, night sweating, dry mouth and throat, dizziness, tinnitus, red tongue with little coating, and fine and rapid pulse.

Pathogenesis of Meridians

Pathogenesis of the meridians refers to the pathological changes caused by direct or indirect affection of pathogenic factors on the meridians.

The pathological changes of meridians are first of all manifested as Excess or Deficiency of Qi and Blood in the meridians. Excess of Qi and Blood in the meridians may cause hyperactivity of the Zang Fu organs that the channel pertain to or connect with, giving rise to disease by disturbing the harmony of the functional activities of the Zang Fu organs and meridians, while Deficiency of Qi and Blood in the meridians may cause disease by giving rise to functional decline of the Zang Fu organs that the meridians pertain to or connect with.

Adverse flow of Qi and Blood in the meridians is also a common pathological changes of meridians disorders, which is usually marked by upward adverse flow of sinking of Qi and Blood due to the adverse ascending or descending movement of Qi of the meridians affecting the normal flow of Qi and Blood. Or the other way round, abnormal flow of Qi and Blood may also cause adverse flow of Qi of the meridians. So there exists a mutual cause-result relationship between them. In most cases, adverse flow of Qi and Blood in the meridians disturbs the communication between Yin and Yang and the ensuing syncope. It may also cause disturbance of the functional activities of the Zang Fu organs related to the meridians, or such symptoms as bleedings.

Slugguish flow of Qi and Blood in the meridians mostly results from invasion of exogenous pathogens or emotional injury which causes unsmooth flow of Qi and the ensuing sluggish flow of Qi and Blood. When Qi and Blood in the meridians flow sluggishly, it may involve the Zang Fu organs related to the meridians, or develop stagnation of Qi or Blood Stasis in a channel.

Exhaustion of Qi and Blood in the meridians is a phenomenon seen at the last gap of life marked by Deficiency and consequent exhaustion of the Qi of meridians and the ensuing exhaustion of Qi and Blood. By observing the manifestations of the exhaustion, one may determine the development and prognosis of a disease.

Pathogenesis of
Zang Fu Organs

This refers to the intrinsic mechanism of the functional disturbance and disharmony between Yin and Yang or Qi and Blood of the Zang Fu organs in the occurrence and development of a disease.

The pathogenesis of Zang Fu rgans occupies an extremely important position in the theory of pathogenesis, because it is the main theoretical basis for Syndrome identification and corresponding treatment in the clinic. The pathogenesis of disturbance of Zang Fu organs mainly includes two types: hyperfunction or hypofunction of the Zang Fu organs and disharmony of the different functional activities, and disturbance of Yin, Yang, Qi and Blood of different Zang Fu organs. The former is what involved in the viscera-state theory, so it is not discussed here.

1. Disturbance of Yin, Yang, Qi and Blood of the Five Zang organs

(1) Disturbance of the Yin, Yang, Qi and Blood of the Heart: The Heart functions to dominate Blood and Blood vessels and con-

trol the mental activities, which result from the harmonious activities of the Yin, Yang, Qi and Blood of the Heart. So disturbance of Yin, Yang, Qi and Blood of the Heart serves as the basis of the Heart diseases.

① Disturbance of the Heart Qi or the Heart Yang: This mainly includes two aspects: Excess of the Heart Yang or Deficiency of the Heart Yang.

Excess of the Heart Yang: Also known as exuberance of the Heart Fire. If it is caused by accumulation of pathogenic Heat in the interior, stagnation of Phlegm Fire in the interior, or the Fire transformed from emotional injury, it is usually excessive in nature, while if it is caused by the relative Excess of the Heart Yang due to over-mental-activities which consumes the Heart Yin and Heart Blood, it is deficient in nature. The Heart Fire of the Excess type and that of the Deficiency type may transform into each other and their influences on the functional activities of the Heart are similar.

Disturbing the Heart spirit, causing Blood Heat and the ensuing accelerated flow of Blood and the up-flaring or downward transmission of the Heart Fire are the main influence of the excessive Heart Fire on the functional activities of the Heart, which are clinically manifested as palpitation, dysphoria, insomnia, dream-disturbed sleep, being talkative, or even mania; palpitation, rapid pulse, red or dark red and prickly tongue, or various kinds of bleeding due to the Blood Heat forcing Blood to extravasate; and erosions or ulcers in the mouth and tongue, burning pain in the tongue tip, dry nose and mouth, scanty dark urine with a burning sensation, respectively.

Deficiency of the Heart Yang or Heart Qi: This includes Deficiency of the Heart Yang and the Deficiency of the Heart Qi, caused mostly by gradual development of the consumption of the Heart Qi or the Heart Yang in chronic disease, or by sudden collapse of the Heart Yang in the critical stage of an acute febrile disease in which the Vital Qi fails in the struggle against the exuberant pathogen. As the Heart Qi Deficiency and the Heart Yang Deficiency share many things in common, they are discussed here collectively.

186

The main influence of the Heart Yang or the Heart Qi on the physiological functions of the Heart mainly includes Deficiency of the Heart spirit and stagnation of pathogenic Cold in the Blood vessels, which are manifested, respectively, as listlessness, slow thinking, delayed response, drowsiness, disinclination to talk, low voice, and aversion to cold, cold limbs, pale and puffy face or dark, dim, blue or purplish face, stuffiness or stabbing pain in the precardiac region, uneven and weak pulse, spontaneous sweating, slow or rapid or knotted and intermittent pulse, or even incessant profuse sweating and prostration.

Deficiency of the Heart Yang often affects the Liver and the Kidney and vice versa.

② Disturbance of the Heart Yin or the Heart Blood: This mainly includes Deficiency of the Heart Yin, consumption of the Heart Blood and the obstruction of the Blood vessels.

Deficiency of the Heart Yin: This is usually caused by over-mental-activities or loss of nourishment in a protracted disease which leads to consumption of the Heart Yin, emotional injury which impairs the Heart Yin, or exuberance of the Heart Fire and the Liver Fire which scorches the Heart Yin. Failure of the deficient Yin to restrict Yang will cause hyperactivity of the Heart Yang and the ensuing production of Fire of Deficiency type in the interior, which is clinically manifested as feverish sensation over the soles, palms and chest, night sweating, restlessness, insomnia, fine and rapid pulse and red tongue.

Consumption of the Heart Blood: This is also known as Deficiency of the Heart Blood, which is mostly caused by loss of Blood, inadequate production of Blood, or consumption of Blood by emotional injury. Blood Deficiency will cause emptiness of the vessels and loss of nourishment of the Heart spirit, so it is clinically manifested as fine and weak pulse, insomnia, dream-disturbed sleep, palpitation, or even fright, panic, distractions, forgetfulness, or a vague mind, pale and lustreless complexion and pale tongue.

Obstruction of Heart vessels: This is a pathological change marked by unsmooth flow of Blood and the ensuing obstruction of

Blood in the Heart vessels, which is usually caused by Deficiency of the Heart Yang or the Heart Qi, stagnation of Cold in the vessels and obstruction of Phlegm. It is usually induced or aggravated by over-fatigue, exposure to cold and emotional disturbance. As a result of Blood obstructing in the Heart vessels or Blood flowing sluggishly, it is usually manifested as stuffiness or pain in the precardiac region and chest, palpitation, or even severe panic with sudden pain in the precardiac region, cold limbs, hidden pulse, sweating and prostration.

(2) Disturbance of the Yin, Yang, Qi and Blood of the Lung: The main functions of the Lung are to dominate Qi and respiration, control dispersion and descension, regulate water metabolism, and meet with all the vessels to assist the flow of Heart Blood. Therefore, disturbance of Yin, Yang, Qi and Blood of the Lung often causes abnormality of respiration, disturbance of the formation of Qi and water metabolism, or abnormal Blood flow as a result of affecting the Heart's function.

The Lung has its own features in physiology, so disturbance of Yin, Yang, Qi and Blood of the Lung is mainly manifested as two types, disturbance of the Lung Qi and that of the Lung Yin.

① Disturbance of the Lung Qi: This consists of disturbance of the Lung Qi's dispersion and descending and Deficiency of the Lung Qi.

Disturbance of the Lung Qi's dispersion and descending: This is mostly caused by attack of exogenous pathogens on the exterior and the Lung, obstruction of Phlegm in the Lung vessels, attack of the Lung by the Fire transformed from excessive ascending of the Liver Qi, Deficiency of the Lung Qi or Deficiency of the Lung Yin.

Failure of the Lung Qi to disperse will cause decline of the respiratory function of the Lung, leading to dyspnea and unsmooth flow of the Lung Qi which, in turns, causes stagnation of the defensive Qi and unconsolidation of the surface of the body, manifested as stuffy nose, frequent sneeze, itchy throat, cough, spontaneous sweating, a tendency to be caught by cold, or night sweating.

Failure of the Lung Qi to descend will give rise to cough with profuse sputum, or chest fullness as a result of decline of the descending and purifying effects of the Lung.

Both failure of the Lung Qi to disperse and that to descend can lead to upward adverse flow of the Lung Qi and influence its regulatory effect on water metabolism, causing oliguria or edema. In the chronic case, it may consume and impair the Lung Qi and the Lung Yin, leading to Deficiency of the Lung Qi or Deficiency of the Lung Yin.

Deficiency of the Lung Qi: This is mostly caused by further development of disturbance of the Lung's dispersion and descending, Qi Deficiency in a chronic disease or consumption of the Lung Qi by over-fatigue. Deficiency of the Lung Qi will give rise to decline of respiratory effect, Deficiency of the defensive Yang and the ensuing unconsolidation of the surface of the body and disturbance of distribution and discharge of the Body Fluid, manifested as shortness of breath, spontaneous sweating, formation of Phlegm or retained fluid or even edema.

② Disturbance of the Lung Yin: This mainly refers to consumption of the Lung Yin and exuberance of Fire due to Lung Yin Deficiency, caused mostly by prolonged attack of pathogenic Dryness or Heat, stagnation of Phlegm and Fire in the Lung, or impairment of the Lung Yin by the Fire transformed from emotional injury. Disturbance of the ascending-descending movements of the Lung Qi due to Lung Dryness and the interior Heat produced by Yin Deficiency impairing the Lung vessels are responsible for various kinds of dry or heat symptoms due to Yin Deficiency, such as dry cough without sputum or with little thick sputum, shortness of breath, hectic fever, night sweating, red cheeks, feverish sensation over the palms, soles and chest, or even cough with blood-stained sputum.

Long-standing Deficiency of Lung Yin often affects the Kidney Yin, leading to Deficiency of both the Lung Yin and the Kidney Yin.

(3) Disturbance of Yin, Yang, Qi and Blood of the Spleen: The main functions of the Spleen are to transform and transport foodstuff, send up nutrients, and keep Blood flowing within vessels. Disturbance of Yin, Yang, Qi and Blood of the Spleen is mainly

189

manifested as Deficiency of the Spleen Qi or the Spleen Yang.

① Disturbance of the Spleen Qi or the Spleen Yang: This includes three types, Deficiency of the Spleen Qi, Deficiency of the Spleen Yang and accumulation of Water Fluid in the Middle Jiao.

Deficiency of the Spleen Qi: Also known as Deficiency of the Qi of the Middle Jiao, which is mostly caused by improper diet causing failure of the Spleen to transform and transport, congenital defect, consumption in chronic diseases, or consumption of the Spleen Qi by over-fatigue. As a result of the Spleen Qi Deficiency and the ensuing failure of the Spleen to transform and transport, patients often present indigestion and tastelessness in the mouth. Due to decline of the function of sending up nutrients, the Stomach will fail to lower down the turbid substance, leading to disturbance of the ascending-descending movements of the Stomach and the Spleen, which is manifested as dizziness, epigastric and abdominal fullness, loose stool or diarrhea. Hypofunction of the Spleen will cause inadeqaute production of Qi and Blood, leading to Deficiency of Qi and Blood in the whole body. If the Spleen fails to keep Blood flowing within vessels, bleeding will ensue. And, if the deficient Spleen Qi is unable to lift, Qi of the Middle Jiao will sink, leading to protracted diarrhea with prolapse of the rectum, or prolapse of other visceral organs.

Deficiency of the Spleen Yang: This mostly arises from the further development of the Spleen Qi Deficiency, or from failure of the Spleen Yang to be warmed in the case of weakness of Fire of Mingmen. Spleen Yang Deficiency produces Cold in the interior, leading to epigastric and abdominal pain with a cold sensation, diarrhea with indigested food, or diarrhea at dawn. Besides, Spleen Yang Deficiency often gives rise to retention of water or fluid in the body as a result of failure of the water to be steamed and transformed.

Accumulation of Water Fluid in the Middle Jiao: This is usually caused by Deficiency of the Spleen Yang and the ensuing failure of the Spleen to transform and transport. Inability of the food to be transformed into nutrients or disturbance of the metabolism of Body Fluid results in retention of water, producing Phlegm or edema. In the case of failure of the deficient Spleen Yang to transform Dampness, exogenous Dampness may invade the human body, leading to combination of the endogenous and the exogenous Dampness and the ensuing accumulation of Dampness in the Middle Jiao which is a Syndrome of Deficiency complicated by Excess. The retained Water Fluid in the Middle Jiao may change into Cold to impair the Spleen, causing exuberance of the Dampness with Yang Deficiency, or into Heat to produce Dampness Heat. The Damp Heat in the Middle Jiao will steam the Liver and the Gallbladder and cause abnormal discharge of bile and Gallbladder Heat, as a result, jaundice marked by yellow coloration over the whole body follows.

② Disturbance of the Spleen Yin: This refers to Deficiency of both the Spleen Qi and the Spleen Yin, caused mostly by failure of the deficient Spleen to transform and transport Body Fluid and the ensuing depletion of the Body Fluid. Deficiency of the Spleen Qi will cause hypofunction of the Spleen, leading to abdominal distention, loose stools and indigestion, while Deficiency of Body Fluid will present such symptoms as dry mouth and throat, red tongue with little coating, etc. Besides, Deficiency of the Spleen Yin is usually complicated by Deficiency of the Stomach Yin, causing upward adverse flow of the Stomach Qi, which is marked by hiccup, or eructation.

(4) Disturbance of Yin, Yang, Qi and Blood of the Liver: The Liver has a mobile and ascending property in physiology and thus bears the name of rigid organ. So, pathogenesis of disturbance of Yin, Yang, Qi and Blood of the Liver is characterized by hyperactivity of the Liver Qi or the Liver Yang, and Deficiency of the Liver Yin and the Liver Blood.

① Disturbance of the Liver Qi or the Liver Yang: This is mainly manifested by exuberance or Excess of the Liver Qi or the Liver Yang, and consists of two main types, stagnation of the Liver Qi and flaring up of the Liver Fire.

Stagnation of the Liver Qi: This is caused mostly by emotional stimuli which leads to mental depression and the ensuing impairment of the Liver. It is marked by distending pain in the affected part. If the stagnated Qi combines with Phlegm or Blood, it may present masses in the diseased area. In the case of the Liver Qi attacking the Spleen and the Stomach transversely, it may cause upward adverse flow of the Stomach Qi, producing eructation, acid regurgitation, or even epigastric pain. And if it attacks the Spleen, it often causes abdominal pain followed by diarrhea.

Flaring up of the Liver Fire: This is usually caused by Fire transformed from the stagnation of the Liver Qi, or impairment of the Liver by sudden rage which again causes upward attack of Qi and Fire, or the Fire transformed from emotional injury. Flaring up of the Liver Fire is in fact the excessive ascending of the Liver Yang, so it is manifested as distending pain in the head, red face and eyes, irritability, sudden deafness or tinnitus. Excessive Liver Fire will consume the Yin Blood, causing exuberance of Fire due to Yin Deficiency. If the Liver Fire scorches the vessels of the Lung or the Stomach, it may lead to hematemesis, epistaxis or coughing blood. And if flaring up of the Liver Fire goes to its extremities, it may cause syncope due to accumulation of Qi and Blood in the upper part.

② Disturbance of the Liver Yin or the Liver Blood: In most cases, the Yin Blood of the Liver tends to be deficient.

Deficiency of the Liver Blood: This arises mostly from loss of Blood, consumption of Blood in a chronic condition, or Deficiency of the Spleen and the Stomach which leads to inadequate production of Qi and Blood. As the Liver is an organ storing Blood, Blood Deficiency involves the Liver first. In the case of Liver Blood Deficiency, the tendons will lose its nourishment, so there is numbness of limbs and difficulty of the limbs to extend and flex. Failure of the deficient Blood to go upward to nourish the head and face will give rise to dizziness, vertigo, dry eyes and blurred vision. And Blood Deficiency is liable to transform into Dryness and produce Wind, leading to stirring of the endogenous Wind of Deficiency type.

Hyperactivity of the Liver: This is mostly caused by Deficiency of the Liver Yin and the resultant excessive ascending of the Liver Yang, or by emotional disturbance which causes upward attack of Qi and Fire and the ensuing hyperactivity of the Liver Yang due to

192

Yin Deficiency. As the Liver Yin and the Kidney Yin communicate with each other, Deficiency of the Kidney Yin also contributes to the hyperactivity of the Liver Yang. Hyperactivity of the Liver Yang is mainly manifested as the symptoms of Excess in the upper part such as dizziness, tinnitus, red face, red eyes with blurred vision, irritability, wiry and rapid pulse. And because of the Deficiency of the Liver Yin and the Kidney Yin, such symptoms as soreness in the loins and weakness of the legs are often detected in the clinic.

Stirring of the Liver Wind: The stirring of the Liver Wind covers a wide range, but that caused by excessive ascending of the Liver Yang due to failure of the deficient Kidney Yin and Liver Yin to restrict is the most commonly encountered. Clinically, it may present tremor of hands and feet, convulsion, or muscular twitching and cramp, involuntary movements of limbs, or even sudden fall with coma and convulsion or tremor.

(5) Disturbance of Yin, Yang, Qi and Blood of the Kidney: The essence Qi in the Kidney is the basis of the Kidney Yin and the Kidney Yang which further serve as the basis of all the Yin and Yang of the human body. Therefore, an evident feature of disturbance of Yin, Yang, Qi and Blood of the Kidney is that only Deficiency of essence Qi of the Kidney is mentioned and no disturbance of Qi and Blood is discussed in theory.

① Deficiency of the Kidney essence or the Kidney Qi: Deficiency of the Kidney essence and the Kidney Qi includes two kinds of pathological changes, Deficiency of the Kidney essence and unconsolidation of the Kidney Qi.

Deficiency of the Kidney essence: This is usually caused by depletion of the kidne essence in the aged, congenital defect, loss of nourishment in chronic disease or improper feeding after birth. Deficiency of the Kidney essence in the infants may delay the development and growth of the infants, that in the adolescence may influence the formation of Tiankui (a substance that can promote maturity of the sexual function) and cause the delayed development of the maturity of the sexual glands. In the middle age, it often leads to early occurrence of senility, decline of the sexual function, manifested as impotence or premature ejaculation. Failure of the Kidney essence to nourish the brain will cause decline of intelligence, slow action, or flaccidity of legs.

Unconsolidation of the Kidney Qi: This is usually caused by inadequate filling of the Kidney essence in the children, reduce of the Kidney essence in the aged, consumption of the Kidney essence due to marrying early or intemperance of the sexual activities, or impairment of the Kidney essence in a prolonged disease. Failure of the deficient Kidney Qi to control will cause the essence Qi in the Kidney to be discharged excessively, manifested as nocturnal emission or loss of control of emission. If the Kidney Qi fails to receive the fresh air inhaled by the Lung, it may result in floating of Qi in the upper part of the body, manifested as dyspnea on slight exertion. Failure of the deficient Kidney Qi to control the defecation and urination may give rise to incontinence of defecation, profuse and clear urine, enuresis, dribbling, or incontinence of urination.

② Disturbance of the Kidney Yin and the Kidney Yang: The Kidney Yin is also known as the genuine Yin, the true Yin, or water of the Mingmen; while the Kidney Yang is also known as the genuine Yang, the true Yang or the Fire of the Mingmen. Disturbance of the Kidney Yin and the Kidney Yang mainly includes two types, Deficiency of the Kidney Yin and insufficiency of the Kidney Yang.

Deficiency of the Kidney Yin: This is mostly caused by consumption of the Kidney Yin in a prolonged disease, Dryness impairing the Kidney essence due to Fire transformed from emotional injury, lingering pathogenic Heat or over-intake of the warm and dry drugs with the action of strengthening Yang, or consumption of the Kidney essence due to excessive sexual intercourse. It may also occur as a result of further development of Yin Deficiency of other organs. Due to Deficiency of the Kidney Yin, the ministerial Fire of Mingmen will be hyperactive, so interior Heat due to Yin Deficiency or flaring up of Fire due to Yin Deficiency follows. Clinically, it is usually manifested as emaciation, soreness and weakness of the loins and knees, feverish sensation over the palms, soles and chest, red cheeks, spontaneous sweating, red tongue with little coating and weak, fine and rapid pulse.

Insufficiency of the Kidney Yang: This is also called decline of the Mingmen Fire which may be either mild or severe in the clinic. In most cases, it arises from consumption of the Kidney Yang by the further development of the Deficiency of the Heart Yang or the Spleen Yang or by excessive sexual intercourse. Yang Deficiency causes generation of Cold of Deficiency type in the interior, so symptoms of Deficiency Cold often oppear. Kidney Yang Deficiency may give rise to impotence, sterility with cold sperm or coldness of the wombs as a result of hypoactivity of the sexual function. Failure of the deficient Kidney Yang to steam will cause disturbance of water metabolism, leading to edema. And, failure of the deficient Kidney Yang to warm the Spleen Yang may result in diarrhea with indigested food or diarrhea at dawn due to inability of the Spleen to transform and transport.

2. Functional disturbance of the Six Fu organs

(1) Functional disturbance of the Gallbladder: This is mainly manifested as disturbance of the bile in its secretion and discharge, which is usually caused by emotional injury which leads to stagnation of the Liver Qi and the ensuing failure of the Liver to discharge, or by steaming of Dampness Heat in the Middle Jiao which obstructs free flow of the Liver Qi. When the bile is unable to be discharged, it may not only aggravate stagnation of the Liver Qi, but also disturb the transforming and transporting effects of the Spleen, or even cause jaundice as a result of overflow of the bile to the skin and muscle.

If the stagnated Heat in the Gallbladder combines with Phlegm, the Phlegm Heat may go upward to attack the Heart, leading to restlessness or insomnia.

(2) Functional disturbance of the Stomach:

① Deficiency of the Stomach Qi: This is mostly caused by long-standing or repeated improper diet, congenital Deficiency of the Stomach or failure of the genuine Qi to restore sooner after a chronic disease. When the Stomach Qi is deficient, it will be unable to perform its receiving and digesting function, leading to poor appetite or

195

even loss of appetite. Failure of the Stomach Qi to descend may cause fullness and distention or mild pain in the epigastric region and abdomen, or even eructation, nausea, hiccup or vomiting in the case of the Stomach Qi flowing upward adversely.

② Deficiency of the Stomach Yin: This usually arises from lingering of pathogenic Heat in the later stage of an febrile disease, or impairment of Yin Fluid in a chronic disease. Generally speaking, when the Stomach Yin is deficient, the receiving and digesting functions of the Stomach will be severely weakened, so there is poor appetite, dry red tongue without coating like a mirror. In the case of the Stomach Qi fails to descend, there is fullness and distention of Deficiency type in the epigastric region and abdomen, frequent nausea or eructation. If the Stomach Qi is exhausted, it may cause erosion in the mouth.

③ The Stomach Cold: This is usually caused by intake of excessive cold food, impairment of the Stomach Yang due to over-use of cold drugs or purgatives, original existence of Cold in the Stomach. The digesting function of the Stomach will decline evidently in the case of the Stomach Cold, so there is indigestion. Besides, Stomach Cold may cause obstruction of Qi or even Blood Stasis and contracture of vessels, leading to severe Stomachache which can be relieved by warmth.

④ The Stomach Heat (Fire): Heat is similar to Fire, exuberant Stomach Heat will become the Stomach Fire if it transforms into Fire due to stagnation and goes upward. In most cases, the Stomach Heat or the Stomach Fire is caused by attack of pathogenic Heat on the Stomach, indulgence in alcohol and preference for hot, acrid, greasy and fatty food which strengthen the Fire and Heat, Fire transformed from stagnation fo Qi, Blood Stasis, Phlegm and retained food, or the transverse attack of the Fire from the Liver and the Gallbladder on the Stomach. The Stomach Heat or Fire will cause hyperactivity of the Stomach, so gastric discomfort and excessive eating occur. The excessive Heat and Fire will also cause impairment of Body Fluid, leading to stagnation of Dry Heat in the interior and failure of the Stomach Qi to descend, so it often presents bitter taste in the mouth, thirst with preference for drinking and constipation, or even develops Deficiency of the Stomach Yin. If the Stomach Fire flares up, it may induce the Stomach Qi to flow upward, leading to nausea or vomiting sour, bitter and yellow fluid. If the Stomach Fire goes upward along its channel, it may result in gum swelling and pain or bleeding gums. And, if it burns the Stomach vessels, it may cause haemetemesis.

(3) Functional disturbance of the Small Intestine: As the physiological functions of the Small Intestine are ascribed to the nutrient-up-sending function of the Spleen and the turbid-down-sending function of the Stomach in the viscera-state theory, most of the functional disturbance of the Small Intestine can be included in the morbid states of the Spleen and the Stomach. Generally speaking, functional disturbance of the Small Intestine in its receiving effect is marked by abdominal pain after eating, diarrhea or vomiting. If the Small Intestine is unable to digest food, it will cause abdominal distention after eating or diarrhea with indigested food. If it fails to separate the nutrients from the waste, it may result in abdominal pain, borborygmus, vomiting with diarrhea, etc.

In addition, Fire of the Small Intestine is often mentioned in the viscera-state theory, which is caused mostly by downward flow of Dampness Heat or the exuberant Heart Fire flowing downward along its channel, manifested as scanty dark urine with a burning sensation during urination, erosion or ulcers in the mouth and red tongue or dribbling of urine with a stabbing pain.

(4) Functional disturbance of the Large Intestine: This is manifested as abnormality of the discharge of faeces. Failure of the Large Intestine to perform its transporting effect may be caused by improper diet, retained food, downward flow of Dampness Heat or Dampness Cold, manifested as diarrhea or loose stool. If the retained food interlocks with Qi and Blood in the Large Intestine, it may give rise to diarrhea with pus and blood and tenesmus. There may appear dry stool or constipation in the case of failure of the Stomach Qi to descend, or failure of the Lung Qi to descend which leads to Dry Heat in the intestine and depletion of the fluid in the in-

197

testine, or in the case of failure of the deficient Yang to move. If the Qi of the Middle Jiao sinks or the Kidney Qi is unable to consolidate, such symptoms as protracted diarrhea, incontinence of defecation or prolapse of the rectum will follow as a result.

(5) Functional disturbance of the Bladder: This is mainly manifested as disturbance of the discharge of urine. The function of the Bladder's storing and discharging urine depends completely on the steaming effect of the Kidney. Therefore, functional disturbance of the Bladder arises from disturbance of the steaming effect of the Kidney. When the steaming effect is disturbed due to excessive pathogen or Deficiency of the Kidney Qi or the Kidney Yang, it may present frequent and urgent urination with turbid urine, dribbling, or difficulty in discharging urine or even retention of urine. On the other hand, if the Kidney fails to store and loses its steaming effect, there may be enuresis and incontinence of urine.

(6) Functional disturbance of the Triple Jiao: The Triple Jiao is the passageway of Qi and Body Fluid. The steaming effect of the Triple Jiao, thus, represents the steaming effect of the whole body. Disturbance of the steaming effect of the Triple Jiao is manifested as two aspects: the disturbance of movement of Qi in the Heart and the Lung, that in the Spleen and the gastrointestinal tract, that in the Liver and the Gallbladder; and that in the Kidney and the Bladder, and the functional disturbance of the Lung, the Spleen and the Kidney in regulating water metabolism, including failure of the Lung Qi to descend in the Upper Jiao, functional disturbance of the Spleen and the Stomach in the Middle Jiao, and the functional disturbance of the Kidney and the Bladder in the Lower Jiao. Therefore, disturbance of the steaming effect of the Triple Jiao is a generalization of the pathological changes involving water metabolism of the whole body.

3. Functional disturbance of the extraordinary organs

The extraordinary organs include the brain, the marrow, the bone, the vessel, the Gallbladder and the uterus. As the Heart dominates vessels, the Kidney is in charge of the bone and marrow, the brain serves as the sea of marrow, the Gallbladder is also one of the Six Fu organs, and the physiological function of the uterus is closely related to the functional activities of the Kidney, the Liver, the Heart and the Spleen, functional disturbance of the extraordinary organs are usually discussed in the pathogenesis of related organs, and thus it is not discussed here.

Principles
for Prevention
and Treatment of
Disease

Prevention

Prevention means to take measures to prevent the occurrence and development of disease. In TCM, prevention of disease has been attached great importance. As early as in *Huang Di Nei Jing* (The Yellow Emperor's Internal Classics), the idea of preventive treatment of disease has been suggested. The preventive treatment of disease consists of two aspects: preventing occurrence of disease and preventing the further development of disease.

1. Preventing occurrence of disease

This indicates that various preventive measures should be taken to prevent occurrence of disease. Invasion of pathogen is a necessary condition for occurrence of disease, while the Deficiency of Vital Qi is the intrinsic basis. So, preventing occurrence of disease should be carried out by strengthening the Vital Qi and preventing invasion of pathogen.

(1) Building up health to enhance the resistant ability of the Vital Qi against disease: The strength of the Vital Qi depends on the constitution, therefore, the key to build up health is to strengthen the constitution, which may be realized by doing the follows:

① Regulating the mental state: TCM holds that emotional activities are closely related to the physiological activities and pathological changes of the human body. An ease mind with pleasant mood can promote flow of Qi, harmonize Qi and Blood and is thus beneficial to one's health, and abnormal emotional stimuli may cause Deficiency of the Vital Qi as well as invasion of pathogen. Therefore, regulation of the mental activities can enhance the resistant ability of the Vital Qi and prevent disease.

② Doing physical exercise: Frequent physical exercise can promote flow of both Qi and Blood, benefit the joints, strength the Vital Qi, and reduce or prevent the occurrence of disease. Such physical fitness exercises as the "Five mimic-animal boxing" created by Hua Tuo, a famous physician in the Han Dynasty, Taiji boxing, Yi Jin Jing (Exercise to Change Your Tendons), etc., can be used to strength the constitution and prevent disease or to treat some chronic diseases as supplements.

③ Living a regular daily life: To adapt the laws of changes of nature, one should arrange well his diet, living, work and rest, so that he can keep fit, be pleasant in spirit and live a long life.

④ Prevention with drugs and vaccination: Proper drugs and artificial immunization are effective measures to prevent disease, especially in the case of spreading of infectious disease.

(2) Preventing invasion of pathogen: Apart from enhancing the resistant ability of the body against disease, one should also prevent invasion of pathogen because pathogen is an inevitable condition for occurrence of disease. Such methods as stressing the sanitary condition, preventing pollution of water source and the food are all effective measures to prevent disease.

2. Preventing the further development of disease

It is the best way to prevent a disease from occurring, but once disease has developed, early diagnosis and early treatment should be conducted as soon as possible to prevent the disease from developing further or transmitting to other organs. After invading the human body, the pathogen may deepen its positions until attacking the Zang Fu organs. So it is imperative to realize the laws of development of disease and the ways the disease transmits in order to diagnose and treat the disease promptly and prevent the further development of the disease. In addition, strengthening the organ that may be transmitted by disease according to the law of disease transmission is also an effective way to prevent the further development of disease.

Principles for Treatment

Principles for treatment in TCM are determined under the guidance of the wholistic concept as well as the principle of Syndrome identification and corresponding treatment. It has a universe significance in guiding selection of the therapeutic methods and giving prescriptions in the clinic.

Both the therapeutic principle and the therapeutic method are of guiding significance for clinical prescription and application of drugs, but they are not the same. The therapeutic principle is a guide to the determination of the therapeutic method, while the therapeutic method is the concrete method to treat disease determined on the basis of the principle. For this reason, any concrete therapeutic method belongs to certain therapeutic principle.

The commonly used therapeutic principles in TCM are as follows:

1. Treating the fundamental cause of disease

This means that one must find out the most basic cause of disease and carry out the treatment aiming at the cause in the treatment of disease. This is a basic principle for Syndrome identification and corresponding treatment.

Diseases may present various kinds of symptoms and signs in their development. But these symptoms and signs are only the manifestations of diseases rather than their essence. So, one must collect, understand and analyze the manifestations comprehensively in order to find out the basic causes of the disease through the manifestations, select correct therapeutic method and achieve satisfactory therapeutic effects. This is just the significance of the principle.

In the process of application of the principle, one must have a good knowledge of the routine treatment, the contrary treatment, treating the superficials and treating the fundamentals.

(1) The routine treatment and the contrary treatment:

① The routine treatment: This is also known as adverse treatment, referring to a therapeutic method by using the drugs opposite to the natures of diseases in the case of agreement of the manifestations with the essence of disease. "Adverse" means that the nature of the selected drugs is opposite to that of the disease. It is carried out by using hot drugs to treat Cold disease, cold drugs to treat Heat disease, tonifying drugs to treat Deficiency disease and purgatives to treat Excess disease based on a correct analysis of the natures of diseases such as Deficiency or Excess, Heat or Cold. The routine treatment is suitable for the diseases, natures of which are coincident with their manifestations. As most diseases seen in the clinic present the manifestations identical with their natures, such as Cold symptoms seen in Cold disease, Heat symptoms seen in Heat disease, Deficiency symptoms seen in Deficiency disease and Excess symptoms seen in Excess disease, the routine treatment is a method that is most frequently adopted in the clinic.

② The contrary treatment: This is a method of treating disease by using the drugs that are identical with the pseudo manifestations of disease in the case of the manifestations being opposite to the nature of disease. As the drugs are identical with the pseudo manifestations of disease which are opposite to its nature, the contrary treatment is still directed at the nature of disease based on the principle of treating the fundamental cause of disease. It is suitable for the treatment of disease with manifestations opposite to its nature.

203

The commonly used contrary treatment methods are as follows:

Treating pseudo Heat with hot drugs: This is a method used to treat disease with pseudo Heat symptoms with cold or cool drugs, suitable for true Cold Syndrome with pseudo Cold symptoms caused by exuberant Cold in the interior keeping Yang Qi staying in the exterior.

Treating pseudo Cold with cold drugs: This is a method used to treat disease with pseudo Cold manifestations with heat or warm drugs, suitable for the disease true Heat in nature with pseudo Cold manifestations caused by Yin being kept in the exterior by the exuberant Yang in the interior.

Treating pseudo obstruction with tonics: This is a method used to treat the disease with pseudo Excess symptoms such as abdominal fullness or distention with tonifying drugs, suitable for the disease Deficiency in nature with pseudo Excess manifestations.

Treating pseudo discharging symptoms with purgatives: This is a method used to treat discharging symptoms with the drugs promoting the discharge. It is suitable for the disease true Excess in nature with pseudo Deficiency manifestations.

(2) Treating the superficial and treating the fundamentals: The "superficial and the fundamental" is a relative concept used to explain the different importance of different contradictions in disease. Generally speaking, the pathogen, compared with the Vital Qi, is the superficial while the Vital Qi is the fundamentals; compared with the symptoms, the cause of disease is the fundamental while the symptoms, the superficial; compared with the secondary disease, the primary disease is the fundamental while the secondary disease, the superficial; and compared with the already existed disease, the newly-developed disease is the superficial while the old disease, the fundamental. As the fundamentals and the superficials of a disease change rapidly and constantly in the process of a complicated and changeable disease, one must pay attentions to the different sequences and importance of these conditions based on the principle of treating the fundamental of disease. For example, in the case of the superficial disease being very urgent, the superficial dis-

ease may cause death or delayed the treatment of the disease as a whole, so the superficial disease should be treated first, and the fundamental disease should be treated later. If both the superficial and the fundamental disease are urgent, they should be treated at the same time.

2. Supporting the Vital Qi and eliminating pathogens

Disease is a process in which the Vital Qi fights against pathogens. The result of the struggle between the Vital Qi and the pathogens determines whether the disease is aggravated or alleviated. Therefore, supporting the Vital Qi and eliminating pathogens form a basic principle of treatment.

The so-called supporting the Vital Qi means to strengthen the Vital Qi or the constitution and to enhance the resistant ability against disease. Eliminating pathogen means to remove the pathogens from the body to stop its damage to the Vital Qi. Supporting the Vital Qi is applicable to the Deficiency disease marked by Deficiency of the Vital Qi with the pathogen being not strong. It is performed by the methods of tonifying the Deficiency, including the acupuncture therapy, Qigong therapy, physical exercise, regulation of mental state and intake of nutritious food. Eliminating pathogens is suitable for the Excess disease marked by exuberance of pathogen with the Vital Qi being not deficient. Usually the method of purging the Excess is adopted in eliminating pathogens, but it should be carried out differently in accordance with the different natures of pathogens and the different locations of disease. Supporting Vital Qi and eliminating pathogens are supplementary to each other and assistant to each other. On one hand, eliminating pathogen can help the Vital Qi to restore, on the other, supporting Vital Qi can help to eliminate the pathogens.

Supporting Vital Qi and eliminating pathogens may be applied simultaneously if supporting Vital Qi does not result in the delayed elimination of pathogens, or if eliminating pathogen leads to no impairment of the Vital Qi in the Syndromes with both exuberance of pathogens and Deficiency of the Vital Qi. If the deficient Vital Qi can still bear the possible damage caused by eliminating pathogens,

205

or if supporting Vital Qi may cause even exuberance of the pathogens, eliminating pathogen should be done first, followed by supporting the Vital Qi. If the Vital Qi is too deficient to bear the damage of eliminating pathogens, it, of course, should be supported first, then followed by eliminating pathogens.

3. Regulating Yin and Yang

The most basic reason for development of disease, in accordance with Yin Yang theory, is the destruction of the harmonious balance between Yin and Yang which is manifested as either Excess of Yin or Yang or Deficiency of Yin or Yang. Therefore, regulating Yin and Yang by reducing the Excess and supplementing the Deficiency to restore the relative balance between Yin and Yang also serves as a basic therapeutic principle that is commonly adopted in the clinic.

The basic method to regulate Yin and Yang is to reduce the Excess and supplement the Deficiency so that the Yin and Yang of the human body can restore their harmony.

Reducing the Excess is suitable for Syndromes marked by Excess of either Yin or Yang. As Excess of Yin or Yang often leads to Deficiency of its opposite, nourishing Yin or supporting Yang should also be considered in the treatment of Excess of Yin or Yang.

Supplementing the Deficiency is suitable for Syndromes marked by either Deficiency of Yin or Deficiency of Yang or both. As Deficiency of Yin or Yang often causes relative hyperactivity of its opposite, nourishing Yin to restrict Yang or supporting Yang to restrict Yin should be used together with the principle of seeking Yang from Yin or seeking Yin from Yang in the treatment of Deficiency of either Yin or Yang.

4. Treatment in accordance with the seasons, geographical conditions and the individual differences

This means that proper therapeutic methods should be taken according to the different seasons, geographical conditions and the difference of the patients in sex, age and constitution in the treatment of disease.

(1) Treatment in accordance with different seasons: This is a principle to determine the treatment in accordance with the different

climates in different seasons. As different climates in different seasons may exert different influences on both the physiological functions and the pathological changes of the human body, a doctor must take the different climates in the different seasons into consideration in treating disease. Generally speaking, the weather changes from warm to hot in the spring and summer, as a result, Yang Qi grows and goes upwards, and the striae of the muscles of the human body opens. In this case, even if a patient is affected by exogenous pathogenic Cold, he should not be treated with drastic diaphoresics of warm and pungent nature lest the excessive discharge of sweating impair Qi and Yin Fluid. In the autumn and winter, however, as the weather changes from cool to cold, Yin becomes exuberant and Yang declines. In this case, the striae of the muscles is closed and Yang Qi of the body goes in the interior, so drugs of cool or cold nature should be used carefully unless severe pathogenic Heat invades the human body, to prevent impairment of Yang Qi. This is what is said in *Liu Yuan Zheng Ji Da Lun* (A Great Treatise on the Six Climates) of *Su Wen* (The Plain Questions): "Drugs with a cold nature should be carefully applied in cold weather, those with a cool nature in cool weather, those with a warm nature in warm weather, and those with a hot nature in hot weather."

(2) Treatment in accordance with different geographical conditions: This is a principle to determine the treatment based on the different geographical conditions in different regions. As a result of the differences in the geographical conditions, the climates and the living habits in different regions, people living in different regions have different physiological features and pathological characteristics. Therefore, treatment should be somewhat different in light of the differences. For example, disease caused by exogenous pathogenic Wind Cold may be treated with drastic diaphoresics of pungent and warm nature such as Ma Huang (Radix Ephedrae) and Gui Zhi (Ramulus Cinnamomi) in the north-west of China where it is very cold; but it can only be treated with less strong diaphoresics of warm and pungent nature such as Jing Jie (Herba Schizonepetae) and Fang Feng (Radix Ledebouriellae) if it is seen in the south-east of China

207

where it is warm and hot.

(3) Treatment in accordance with individual difference : This is a principle to determine treatment in accordance with the differences of different patients in age, sex, constitution and living habits.

Patients of different ages have different physiological states and different Qi and Blood, so they should be treated differently. The aged people, for example, have a declined vitality and their Qi and Blood are deficient, so they are liable to be affected by Deficiency disease or the Excess disease complicated by Deficiency, and therefore tonifying method is more frequently adopted and even if they suffer from an Excess Syndrome, dosage of the purgative drugs should be less than that in young people. In the children, disease tends to change rapidly, because the children are full of life, their Qi and Blood are not well supplemented and their Zang Fu organs are still tender. So in the treatment of children's diseases, drastic purgatives should be avoided, tonics should be applied carefully and the dosage of the drugs applied should be less.

Male is different from female, so they have different physiological features. In the treatment of disease, such features of the female as menstruation, leukorrhea, pregnancy and delivery must be fully considered. During the pregnancy, drastic purgatives, drugs that eliminating Blood Stasis, drugs with a smooth or aromatic nature or the toxic drugs that may cause miscarriage should not be used. And, after delivery, drugs tonifying Qi and Blood as well as those eliminating the lochia should be more adopted.

The constitutions of different people vary in strong, weak, cold or heat, so they should be treated differently. For those with a Yang Excess or Yin Deficiency constitution, warm or hot drugs should be carefully used, and for those with a Yang Deficiency or Yin Excess constitution, drugs of cool or cold nature that may impair Yang Qi should be avoided unless necessary.

Besides, the different past history of disease, the different emotional states and the different living habits of patients should be well considered in the treatment of disease.

Treatment in accordance with the different seasonal conditions, the different geographical conditions and the individual differences shows that the application of the wholistic concept and the principle of Syndrome identification and corresponding treatment is flexible. Only the treatment is carried out in accordance with the different seasonal conditions, the different geographical conditions and the individual difference, better therapeutic effects can be obtained.

中医基础

编　　著　欧阳兵
　　　　　顾　真
译　　者　路玉滨
责任编辑　仲彭军

*

山东科学技术出版社出版
济南市玉函路 16 号　邮政编码　250002
山东德州新华印刷厂印刷
中国国际图书贸易总公司发行
中国北京车公庄西路 35 号
北京邮政信箱第 399 号　邮政编码　100044

*

1996 年(大 32 开)　1 版 1 次
ISBN 7－5331－1843－X
R・535
07200
14－E－3028P